Preface

The papers contained in this volume represent a wide range of interests in the area of psychosocial oncology and are the proceedings of two meetings organized by the British Psychosocial Oncology Group during 1985 and 1986. Much of the work described is new and currently in progress. Thus the book constitutes an important source of up to date research findings and issues being examined by U.K. and European workers. The fact that many papers are multi-disciplinary in content enhances their usefulness in an area of increasing interest: the psychosocial impact of cancer diagnosis and treatment.

Maggie Watson
Steven Greer
Chris Thomas

PSYCHOSOCIAL ONCOLOGY

Proceedings of the Second and Third meetings
of the British Psychosocial Oncology Group
London and Leicester, 1985 and 1986

M. WATSON and S. GREER

Cancer Research Campaign
Psychological Medicine Group
The Royal Marsden Hospital Sutton, Surrey,UK

and

C. THOMAS

Department of Psychiatry
Leicester General Hospital, Leicester, U.K.

PERGAMON PRESS

OXFORD · NEW YORK · BEIJING · FRANKFURT
SÃO PAULO · SYDNEY · TOKYO · TORONTO

U.K.	Pergamon Press, Headington Hill Hall, Oxford OX3 0BW, England
U.S.A.	Pergamon Press, Maxwell House, Fairview Park, Elmsford, New York 10523, U.S.A.
PEOPLE'S REPUBLIC OF CHINA	Pergamon Press, Room 4037, Qianmen Hotel, Beijing, People's Republic of China
FEDERAL REPUBLIC OF GERMANY	Pergamon Press, Hammerweg 6, D-6242 Kronberg, Federal Republic of Germany
BRAZIL	Pergamon Editora, Rua Eça de Queiros, 346, CEP 04011, Paraiso, São Paulo, Brazil
AUSTRALIA	Pergamon Press Australia, P.O. Box 544, Potts Point, N.S.W. 2011, Australia
JAPAN	Pergamon Press, 8th Floor, Matsuoka Central Building, 1-7-1 Nishishinjuku, Shinjuku-ku, Tokyo 160, Japan
CANADA	Pergamon Press Canada, Suite No. 271, 253 College Street, Toronto, Ontario, Canada M5T 1R5

First edition 1988

Library of Congress Cataloging in Publication Data
British Psychosocial Oncology Group. Conference
(2nd : 1985 : London, England)
Psychosocial oncology
(BPOG: 2)
1. Cancer – Psychological aspects – Congresses.
2. Cancer – Social aspects – Congresses. I. Watson, M. II. Greer, S. (Steven) III. Thomas, C. IV. British Psychosocial Oncology Group. Conference (3rd : 1986 : Leicester, Leicestershire) V. Title. VI. Series: BPOG (Series) ; 2, [DNLM: 1. Neoplasms – psychology – congresses. W3 BR456 2nd–3rd 1985–86p / QZ 200 B8648 1985–86p]
RC262.B755 1985   616.99'4'0019   87-21697

British Library Cataloguing in Publication Data
Psychosocial oncology : proceedings of the second and third meetings of the British Psychosocial Oncology Group, London & Leicester, 1985 and 1986.
1. Cancer – Psychological aspects 2. Cancer – Social aspects
I. British Psychosocial Oncology Group. *(Conference 2nd : 1985 : London)* II. British Psychosocial Oncology Group. *(Conference : 3rd : 1986 : Leicester)*
III. Watson, M. IV. Greer, S. V. Thomas, C.
616.99'4'0019   RC262

ISBN 0–08–035745–8

Pa___ 3933 (2) /36. 3.91

Printed in Great Britain by A. Wheaton & Co. Ltd., Exeter

Contents

viii   *Contents*

Contents ix

enthusiastic

List of Contributors*

AHMEDZAI, S. The Leicestershire Hospice, Groby Road, Leicester, U.K.

ASHCROFT, J. A. School of Psychology, Lancashire Polytechnic, Preston, U.K.

BOS, G., Department of Obstetrics and Gynaecology, University Hospital, Rijnsburgweg 10, Leiden, The Netherlands.

BURTON, M. V. Department of Psychology, Walsgrave Hospital, Walsgrave, Coventry, U.K.

CHARLTON, A. Cancer Research Campaign Education and Child Studies Research Group, Christie Hospital, Wilmslow Road, Manchester, U.K.

CLACEY, R. Mendip Hospital, Wells, Somerset, U.K.

COOPER, A. F. Leverndale Hospital, Crookston Road, Glasgow, U.K.

DAWSON, A. A. Department of Medicine, Aberdeen Royal Infirmary, Aberdeen, U.K.

GOLDIE, L. The Royal Marsden Hospital, Fulham Road, London, U.K.

GREER, S. Cancer Research Campaign Psychological Medicine Research Group, The Royal Marsden Hospital, Downs Road, Sutton, U.K.

DE HAES, J. C. J. M. Instituut voor Sociale Geneeskunde, Wassenaarseweg 62, Leiden, The Netherlands.

HUGHES, J. Department of Psychiatry, Royal South Hants Hospital, Southampton, U.K.

HUGHSON, A. V. M. University Department of Psychological Medicine, Glasgow, U.K.

JONES, D. R. Department of Clinical Epidemiology and Social Medicine, St. George's Hospital Medical School, Cranmer Terrace, London, U.K.

KURTZ, Z. Department of Paediatric Epidemiology, Institute of Child Health, London, U.K.

LEE, D. Medical School, University of Southampton, U.K.

LEINSTER, S. J. Department of Surgery, University of Liverpool, U.K.

LUNT, B. Cancer Care Research Unit, Royal South Hants Hospital, Southampton U.K.

MORTON, A. Department of Respiratory Medicine, Royal Infirmary, Glasgow, U.K.

MOSS, G. Avon Child and Family Guidance Service, Coleridge Vale Road South, Clevedon, Avon, U.K.

MOYNIHAN, C. Department of Radiotherapy, The Royal Marsden Hospital, Downs Road, Sutton, Surrey, U.K.

OWENS, R. G. Sub-Department of Clinical Psychology, University of Liverpool, Liverpool, U.K.

PARKER, R. W., Walsgrave Hospital, Walsgrave, Coventry, U.K.

PEARSON, H. Department of Surgery, Leicester Royal Infirmary, Leicester, U.K.

PECKHAM, M. Department of Radiotherapy, The Royal Marsden Hospital, Downs Road, Sutton, Surrey, U.K.

POSNER, T. Policy Studies Institute, 100, Park Village East, London, U.K.

POT-MEES, C. Department of Child Psychiatry, Westminster Children's Hospital, London, U.K.

RAMIREZ, A. J. United Medical and Dental Schools, Guy's Hospital, London, U.K.

RATCLIFFE, M. A. Department of Medicine, Aberdeen Royal Infirmary, U.K.

REID, J. T. Department of Respiratory Medicine, Royal Infirmary, Glasgow, U.K.

SLADE, P. D. Sub-Department of Clinical Psychology, University of Liverpool, U.K.

STEVENSON, R. D. Department of Respiratory Medicine, Royal Infirmary, Glasgow, U.K.

THOMAS, C. Department of Psychiatry, Leicester General Hospital, Leicester, U.K.

WARING, H. Department of Mental Health, University of Aberdeen, Aberdeen, U.K.

WILKINSON, S. Department of Nursing, University of Manchester, Oxford Road, U.K.

WILLIAMS, C. J. Cancer Research Campaign, Wessex Medical Oncology Unit, University of Southampton, U.K.

YARDLEY, J. Cancer Care Research Unit, Royal South Hants Hospital, Southampton, U.K.

*Requests for reprints should be made directly to the senior authors of individual papers.

PART ONE

Childhood Cancer

Psychological Problems of Children with Bone Marrow Transplantation

CARIEN POT-MEES

ABSTRACT

Bone marrow transplantation (BMT) is now being used as treatment for a wide variety of life-threatening diseases in children, such as leukaemia, neuroblastoma, genetic disorders and immune deficiencies. The treatment, which can be lethal in itself, involves a variety of stressful aspects for the child and the entire family. A systematic prospective study with 75 patients is currently in progress, looking at the long-term effects of BMT in children. The method of this study is discussed and some preliminary observations on patients and families coping are reported. It is advocated that psychological care should be addressed during the entire treatment process and should include siblings and parents as well as patients.

INTRODUCTION

Due to the continuing progress in the medical sciences, to date children with chronic and/or fatal diseases are faced with a longer period of survival and a higher chance of ultimate disease-free survival. We are therefore now in the situation where issues of a non-medical nature can be addressed, such as the psychological well-being of patients and families and the occurrence of possible post-treatment disturbance. Over recent years several studies have enabled us to learn more about the psychological effects of childhood cancer. It is suggested that there are possible effects on the development of personality and cognitive abilities in the child (Lansky and Gendel, 1978; Jannoun, 1983), on the child's relationship with family members and peer group (Kalnins et al., 1980) and on the school adjustment and attainments (Lansky et al., 1984). An aspect which is now receiving more attention is the re-integration of the child into "normal life" and the planning of services, which should help the child and family in their long-term adjustment (Van Eys, 1977; Kagen-Goodheart, 1977; Koocher et al., 1980).

Psychosocial research in the area of chronic illness in childhood should be focused on the following three questions:

(i) What are the psychosocial needs of the child and family during the *entire* process of illness and treatment?
(ii) What are the needs of the child and family when ultimate survival has been reached?

3

(iii) What are the implications for the planning of psychosocial and therapeutic services during and after the process of illness and treatment?

We need to use systematic research to answer the above questions and to devise ways of intervention which are focused on the individual needs of patients and families (Spinetta, 1982).

An example of an intrusive, but potentially curable treatment for children is bone marrow transplantation (BMT). This paper first discusses some of the medical and psychological stressors related to this type of treatment. Then it reports the method of a current study, looking at the long term effects of BMT in children. Finally it describes some preliminary observations on the coping of patients and families during the BMT treatment.

Bone marrow transplantation

BMT is being used for treatment of the following diseases in childhood: leukaemia, immune deficiency states, severe aplastic anaemia, other serious haemotological disorders (thalassaemia-B major, Fanconi's anaemia) and certain genetic and metabolic disorders (Gauchers disease, Hurlers syndrome, Hunters syndrome). The latter three groups can suffer from mental and/or physical retardation caused by their illness. "Allogeneic" BMT consists of the transference of bone marrow cells, which are obtained from a healthy immunologically compatible donor and transfused into the bloodstream of the recipient.

Donors consist of the siblings or relatives of the child and in some cases unrelated donors are selected. The donor, who requires a hospitalization of 2-3 days (including a general anaesthetic) suffers only from short term complaints such as pain and soreness in the hips. The literature suggests that donors can suffer from psychological problems afterwards (Wiley *et al.*,1984). A second form is "autologous" BMT, which is being used when no donor can be found. The patient's bone marrow is taken out and after the marrow has been treated and the patient has received chemotherapy, it is then given back to him. It is difficult to give an overall figure for survival of the treatment, as this can differ according to type of disease, stage of disease and compatibility of the donor. The literature quotes a general survival rate of approximately 50–70%, with a wide differentiation for the individual disorders treated (Kamani and August, 1984). The major problems encountered with BMT at the moment are those of: availability of suitable donors, graft rejection, graft-vs-host disease (GVHD) and death from GVHD, infections or subsequent complications.

BMT treatment requires a lengthy and often traumatic hospital stay for the child and usually one parent, which can take 3–4 months. For part of this time the children undergo isolation in a sterile environment, under conditions of reverse barrier nursing (for an average period of 4–8 weeks). This is carried out in a Laminair Airflow® cubicle or in ordinary cubicles with sterile precautions. The child is not allowed to leave his room at any time and visitors entering the room have to gown up and wear a mask, hat and gloves. Daily medical care and drug management is intrusive and lengthy, affecting the appearance (hair loss), appetite and sometimes the neurological functioning of the patients. For most patients treatment includes total body irradiation which can cause lethargy in the short term and possible cognitive impairment in the long term (Gottschalk *et al.*, 1982 Tamarott *et al.*, 1982). Daily procedures are carried out to maintain strict cleanliness such as mouthwash and total body wash with a Hibiscrub® detergent.

It is only recently that survival rates have been increasing and more children are going home to lead a normal life again. It is understandable that there is concern about the possible psychological impact of the treatment on the child, as well as his family. Several questions can be raised: Is it ethically justifiable to submit children to this treatment? What are the long term implications of the isolation and drug management? How is the patient's quality of life afterwards: is he able to readjust to a "normal life" again? What are the effects on the siblings and the rest of the family?

It is clear that BMT involves complex psychological aspects not only for the child but also for the siblings (the donors and non-donors) and the parents. To date, most of the literature has consisted of descriptive reactions of children and families during and after the treatment (Farkas Patenaude *et al.*, 1977; Farkas Patenaude, 1982; Freund & Siegal, 1986; Kamphuis, 1979; Popkin and Moldow, 1977). Systematic research is needed in order to measure the impact of the procedure and the nature of any possible resulting disturbance. Consequently one will be able to plan adequate therapeutic input for patients and families before, during and after the treatment process.

THE STUDY: AIMS, SUBJECTS AND METHOD

A prospective study was set up to identify the problems of BMT patients and their families before, during and after the treatment process. The study had the following aims:

(i)   to identify the effects of the BMT treatment on the psychological functioning of child and family;

(ii)   to analyze the nature of the positive and negative effects; and

(iii)   to consider the implications for the future management of patients, including the provision of psychological support.

The theory of stress and coping as developed by Lazarus (1966) and Cox (1978) is used in the study as a theoretical framework to look at the individual differences between the patients and their ways of coping.

Prior to the main data collection, which started in 1984 and lasted for the main part of 1987, a pilot study was carried out with 15 patients. Findings are reported elsewhere (Pot-Mees and Zeitlin, 1987). Data collection and follow up appointments are still in progress and therefore we cannot provide any systematic findings at the moment. Preliminary findings and observations on the adjustment of those patients are available and will be presented in the latter part of the paper. It should be noted that they are mainly based on the author's observations.

The study consisted of three groups, which were followed longitudinally and cross-sectionally. The experimental group contained 75 children, between 0 and 16 years of age, who received an allogeneic or autologous BMT for the disorders described above. They and their families were selected from the following four BMT centres in London: Westminster Children's Hospital, Hammersmith Hospital, The Hospital for Sick Children in Great Ormond Street and The Royal Marsden Hospital.

No strict control groups were used as this would imply the random allocation to a life-saving treatment. It was decided to use 'reference groups' instead. The first reference group consisted of 75 children undergoing another stressful hospital intervention, namely open heart surgery. The second reference group consisted of 75 normally healthy children, without any medical problem, selected from the Registry of the Dental Outpatients Clinic and local Health Centres. The three groups were matched for age, sex and IQ and in addition the experimental and second reference group were also matched for social class.

The BMT patients and their families were tested before the start of the BMT procedure and again at 6 and 12 months afterwards. The reference groups were tested respectively (1) before start of surgery and (2) at a certain point in time and again 12 months later.

Areas of assessment for the child included: cognitive functioning, school attainments, behaviour at home and at school and self-perception. Parents were assessed with regard to their mental state, marital relationship, coping skills, social support system and locus of control. Siblings, inclusive of the donors and non-donors, were assessed with regard to their behaviour at home and at school. The assessment consisted of a psychological testing of the child and two interviews with the parents, held at each test occasion.[1]

PRELIMINARY OBSERVATIONS: COPING OF PATIENTS AND FAMILIES DURING BMT TREATMENT

One can differentiate between the following three stages in the bone marrow transplant procedure; (i) the stage pre-transplant, (ii) the

---

[1]Details of the test instruments are not reported here, but information can be obtained from the author.

transplant procedure and subsequent hospitalization and, (iii) the stage after the patient has been discharged from hospital.

(i) Pretransplant stage

This starts at the moment when the possibility of BMT treatment is offered. There are two main phases:

(a) *Tissue typing.* In order to detect the best possible match for the child, blood samples are taken from all family members including the siblings. On the surface this particular event does not seem to be very intrusive and is treated more or less as an administrational aspect by the hospital. However, it appears to create feelings of anxiety for parents and siblings involved. Parents know that obtaining a fully matched donor, only a 1 in 4 chance, is the best opportunity for a cure. Siblings, "normally" anxious about having a blood test, are often aware of the importance of them being a perfect match for their sick brother or sister. This can create additional pressure. In some cases it is necessary to screen the extended family such as uncles and aunts. This can in itself cause pressure, when relationships in the family have previously been cut off or disturbed but now need to be restored because of the search for a possible donor.

(b) *Waiting for admission.* When a donor has been found and a transplant has been planned, the family usually has a time of waiting before admission to the hospital. This time of waiting can range from only a few days (in acute cases, such as immune deficiencies or aplastic anaemia) to a year or more. At this stage communication between the hospital and family is of great importance.

At this time the parents' feelings of hope are predominating. They do experience ambivalence about their decision for treatment, however, and some report that the longer the time of waiting, the more doubtful they feel about their decision for a BMT.

Parents tend to re-organize their lives around the possible date of admission. Whenever the date is postponed, changed or still uncertain, this can have serious implications for events planned in the family such as holidays, Christmas celebrations, etc. Parents often suffer from feelings of frustration when the child cannot be admitted in the near future and prolonged waiting makes them worry that time is "running out".

The patient's adjustment and well-being during the waiting time is related to age, disease and medical condition (Pot-Mees *et al.*, 1987). For example, most children suffering from genetic disorders are usually leading a relatively normal life at home, with, for the older ones, some form of schooling. On the contrary most patients with lymphoma or leukaemia spend their time before BMT in the hospital undergoing maintenance or prophylactic treatment.

Siblings also experience feelings of ambivalence. In their case this is related to their donorship, as also reported by Farkas Patenaude *et al.* (1977). The donor siblings experience feelings of pride on one side, as if they were "chosen" to fulfill this role. On the other hand they have fears about failing in their mission. The non-donor siblings experience feelings of relief, as they do not have to undergo the hospitalization. However, they can easily feel left out and jealous because they are not part of the hospital situation in which patient, parents and donor are involved.

(ii) Stage of BMT

When finally the admission for BMT takes place, this is initially experienced as relief, especially by the parents. One can also divide this stage into two main phases: (a) the preparation, (b) start of isolation and transplant.

(a) *Preparation*. This usually takes 1-2 weeks. Several factors influence the child's adjustment at this stage. Firstly, whether he has been a patient on this ward before, or has come to an entirely new ward with all new faces. Secondly, his experience of previous hospitalizations, their duration and intensity. Also factors such as age, disease and family support play an important role in his adjustment. Children who are new to the ward usually show withdrawn behaviour for the first days, tend to feel insecure in a new environment and need time for adjustment. They easily pick up the anxieties which are present in their parents.

Parents are at this time usually in a stage of "dreaming" especially when they have experienced a long period of waiting and uncertainty. Feelings of excitement and unrealistic expectations about the coming treatment do gradually fade when they meet other patients on the ward and are faced with the actual situation. When preparation, documentation and interviews with the medical staff have not been taking place properly before this admission, parents are confronted with an enormous amount of new information. In most cases, as mentioned before, one parent, usually the mother is admitted to the hospital with the child. This has implications for all the members of the family and makes it necessary for them to get used to new roles. The resident parent in hospital is confronted with feelings of sole responsibility for the medical care of the child, while the parent staying behind has to face responsibility for running the whole household, as well as earning a living in most cases. Siblings are looked after either by the parent at home or by relatives or friends. Whether the rest of the family can stay intact will have an influence on how siblings cope with the situation. However, in most cases siblings experience a prolonged absence from their mother, which can lead to the onset of later behavioural and emotional problems.

(b) *Start of isolation and transplant.* The start of the isolation procedures is often experienced by family as well as staff as the point of "no return". The transplant itself is, in fact, nothing more than a blood transfusion and can be an anticlimax for parent and child who have been looking forward to this day for such a long time. The physical condition of the child and the effects of the new graft influence his mental state during the subsequent hospitalization. It is a common finding (Farkas Patenaude *et al.*, 1977; Kamphuis, 1979, Pot-Mees *et al.*, 1987) that the children tend to show periods of depression and anxiety related to the isolation procedures. Issues of control play an important role, with periodic refusal to take medicine or food. Children tend to experience boredom and frustration the longer the isolation procedures take. When children are physically deteriorating they show further withdrawal and regression. There is a large group of children who never return home and die in hospital as a result of the BMT procedure.

Due to the intensity of the hospital situation, parents tend to experience feelings of claustrophobia and hospitalization themselves, and suffer from mental and physical fatigue which become more intense when the hospitalization is prolonged. The family members at home have to deal with pressures from both inside as well as outside the family. The social environment can provide a useful social support system, but also an extra burden.

(iii) Post transplant stage.

The patient's discharge from the hospital means in most cases, in Britain, a direct re-entry into the home situation. Again one can notice feelings of ambivalence within the child, parents and siblings. The child is looking forward to being back at home and has fantasies about the newly acquired freedom and "normality". On the other hand, because of his previous protected state he can be more anxious about a new confrontation with the outside world and he may feel reluctant to leave behind the special position acquired during his hospital stay. He needs to "re-establish" a place at home and suddenly needs to compete with siblings for parental attention.

Parents' feeling of ambivalence are centred around the following issues. They are losing the direct support of hospital staff and friends and are faced with sole responsibility for medication and care of the child. This creates feelings of insecurity and isolation. On the other hand, they look forward to regaining their privacy and re-establishing a normal life again. This is often not easy as they are mentally and physically very tired at a time when they also give extra attention to the other children and their partner. The first weeks at home are therefore usually a very strained time, and in some ways an anticlimax for all members of the family. Patient's isolation from public places is still required until 6 months post-BMT, which adds a strain to the family routine and restricts family members' excursions.

Siblings also have their ambivalent reaction. They look forward to a reunion of the family and the presence of the absent parent. It also means that they have to give up the extra freedom which they acquired during the previous months. Feelings of resentment towards the patient and the absent parent can occur and siblings can easily feel rejected. At this time siblings are often made to feel responsible for care of the returning patient and this can prevent them from expressing their anger or jealousy in a "normal way". It depends on the patient's state of recovery as well as the coping of family members whether they are able to re-adjust to a normal life in a relatively short period or not. In general it tends to take approximately a year before normality has returned to the family. However, the fear that the disease can reoccur, particularly in patients with leukaemia, is present for a much longer period. This fear will only gradually diminish, and depends on the duration and course of the patient's recovery.

CONCLUSIONS

This paper describes a current study into the psychological implications of BMT and gives some preliminary observations by the author.

The following aspects have become clear while carrying out the study:

1. BMT is an intervention with implications not only for the child, but for the entire family unit. This implies that the psychological care given during the treatment process should be focused on child and family members and professionals should be aware of the possible impact on siblings and parents.

The fact that the child suffers from a potentially fatal disorder is likely to put a strain on the child and family. BMT treatment usually contains the only possibility for cure, but at the same time it is a life-threatening intervention in itself. Parents have to balance the immediate risks of submitting their child to a life-threatening procedure, which can result in possible death, against the long term prospect of losing their child anyway. As reported before (Pot-Mees *et al.*, 1986), parents reported a high incidence of depression and distress during the stage before BMT. This is not surprising and could be expected, given the stressful situation they are facing. However, it also means that parents are unlikely to take in all the information given to them. Families would benefit from repeated information and adequate communication with the hospital during the stage of waiting for the transplant.

2. The treatment process of BMT consists of different stages and possible effects on patient and family are not necessarily restricted to

the period in hospital. It seems appropriate to differentiate between effects before, during and after the treatment process and to identify at each stage the problems and needs of child and family.

The reported observations suggest that there may be long term effects related to BMT. The final results of the current study, which are expected in Autumn 1987, will hopefully shed further light on this.

ACKNOWLEDGEMENTS

The study on which this paper is based is funded by the Cancer Research Campaign. The author is grateful for the assistance of Dr. H. Zeitlin, J. Wray and S. Kelly at the Department of Child Psychiatry, Westminster Children's Hospital and for the cooperation of children, families and staff in the four BMT Centres.

REFERENCES

Cox, T. (1978) *Stress.* Macmillan, London.

Farkas Patenaude, A., Szymanski, L. and Rappeport, J. (1977) Psychological costs of bone marrow transplantation in children. *Am. J. Orthopsychiat.* **49**(3), 409–422.

Farkas Patenaude, A. (1982) Surviving bone marrow transplantation: the patient in the other bed. *Ann. Intern. Med.* 97, 915–918.

Freund, B. L. and Siegel, K. (1986) Problems in transition following bone marrow transplantation: psychosocial aspects. *Am. J. Orthopsychiat.* **56**(2), 244–252.

Gottschalk, Louis A., Kunkel, R., Wohl, T. H., Saenger, E. L. and Winget, C. N. (1982) Total and half body irradiation. *Arch. Gen. Psychiat.* **21**, 574–850.

Jannoun, L. (1983) Are cognitive and educational development affected by age at which prophylactic therapy is given in acute lymphoblastic leukemia? *Arch. Dis. Child.* **58**, 953–958.

Kagen-Goodheart, L. (1977) Reentry: living with childhood cancer. *Health and Soc. Work.* **1**, 71-87.

Kalnins, I. V., Churchill, M. P. and Terry, G. E. (1980) Concurrent stresses in families with a leukaemic child. *J. Pediat. Psychol.* **5**, 81–92.

Kamani, N. and August, C. S. (1984) Bone marrow transplantation: problems and prospects. *Med. Clin. North Am.* **68**(3), 657–674.

Kamphuis, R. P. (1979) Psychological and ethical considerations in the use of germ-free treatment. *Clin. Exp. Gnotobiot.* **361** *Bakt. Suppl.* 7.

Koocher, G. P., O'Malley, J. E., Gogan, J. L., Foster, D. J. (1980) Psychological adjustment among pediatric cancer survivors. *J. Child Psychol. Psychiat.* **21**, 163–173.

Lansky, S. B. and Gendel, M. (1978) Symbiotic regressive behavior patterns in childhood malignancy. *Clin. Paediat.* **17**, 133–138.

Lansky, S. B., Cairns, N. U., Lansky, L. L., Cairns, G. F., Stephenson, L. and Garin, G (1984) Central nervous system prophylaxis: studies showing impairment in verbal skills and academic achievement. *Am. J. Pediat. Hematol./Oncol.* **5**, 183–190.

Lazarus, R. S. (1966) *Psychological Stress and the Coping Process.* McGraw-Hill, New York.

Popkin, M. K. and Moldow, C. F. (1977) Stressors and responses during bone marrow transplantation. *Arch. Intern. Med.,* **137**.

Pot-Mees, C., Wray, J. and Zeitlin, H. (1986) Psychosocial issues in paediatric bone marrow transplantation. *Bone Marrow Transplantation,* **1**, Suppl. 1, 220.

Pot-Mees, C., Wray, J., Zeitlin, H. (1987) The psychosocial state of 75 paediatric patients and their families when entering the BMT treatment. *Bone Marrow Transplantation,* **2**, Suppl., 247.

Pot-Mees, C. and Zeitlin, H. (1987) Psychosocial consequences of bone marrow transplantation in children: A preliminary communication. *J. Psychosoc. Oncol.* **5**, 2.

Spinetta J.J. (1982) Behavioral and psychological research in childhood cancer. *Cancer suppl.* **50**, 1939-1943.

Tamaroff, M., Miller, D. R., Murphy, M. L., Salwen, R., Ghavimi, F. and Nir, Y. (1982) Immediate and long-term posttherapy neuropsychologic performance in children with acute lymphoblastic leukemia treated without central nervous system radiation. *J. Pediat.* **101**(4), 524–529.

Van Eys, J. (1977) *The Truly Cured Child.* University Park Press, Baltimore.

Wiley, F. M., Lindamood, M. M. and Pfefferbaum-Levine, B. (1984) Donor–patient relationship in pediatric bone marrow transplantation. *Assoc. Pediat. Oncol. Nurs.* **I**(3), 8–14

A Case Study of Multiple Stressors and Coping in a Child Treated for Leukaemia

GEOFFREY MOSS

ABSTRACT

Research on children's reactions to stressful events is a relatively neglected area. There are important developmental and social differences in the ways children appraise and cope with stress compared with adults.

A single case study of a 14-year-old boy treated for leukaemia describes the multiple stressors that acted upon him; at an organic, neurological level, at a personal, psychological level and at a family, social level. His coping strategies drew upon cognitive, emotional and behavioural responses in a free-ranging manner suggesting those distinctions may be arbitrary. The concept of emotion – or problem-focused coping strategies is questioned. In the case of children and young people, stress and coping must take account of their social as well as psychological systems.

Despite its increasing usage in psychological studies, the concept of "stress" continues to be criticized because of the imprecision of the term and the variety of meanings ascribed to it by researchers. As a result attention has started to shift away from attempts to create a general theory of stress, and to focus instead on identifying critical parameters that might characterize specific stress situations. However, research on the reactions of children to stressful events is still a relatively neglected area in comparison to the many studies of adults (Garmezy and Rutter, 1983).

There are important differences between adults and children in the context of their reactions to stressful events. Children are themselves more in the process of change and are likely to be interacting with environments that are more variable than are adults. Equally they may be less able than adults to ascertain to what extent environmental conditions and sudden dramatic life changes are relevant factors in their ability to cope; they are likely to be less able to judge which situations are potentially threatening. While their threat appraisal processes may be less sophisticated than adults, they will tend, even in late adolescence, to appraise and utilize their adult caretakers as part of their coping strategies. Children and young people will use the social support system of their family as an integral part of their efforts to adapt and cope. A

13

study of child stress and coping, then, must adopt a systemic perspective that incorporates the child's social ecology. The interaction of these systems, from the organic to the psychological to the social, in respect of the stresses upon them and the coping responses produced by them, may be shown in a case study of one child treated for leukaemia.

'Paul' a 14-year-old, was the elder of two sons of well-educated professional parents.

We met shortly after his admission to the Royal Hospital for Sick Children, Bristol. I was able to interview him and his parents then as part of a study currently being conducted by the paediatric oncology department into the psychological stresses of children receiving various chemotherapy treatments. Paul was diagnosed as suffering from stem cell leukaemia, and he was to be treated according to the U.K.A.L.L. X (Regimen D) protocol. This would have meant his receiving an induction phase of chemotherapy for the first 4 weeks, leading into early intensification at week five, radiotherapy from weeks nine to eleven, and late intensification at week twenty. The physical stresses of receiving cytotoxic drugs can be severe, disrupting the body's homeostatic systems and suppressing its immune system.

During the early stages of Paul's induction treatment he developed diabetes. By the eighth day he was suffering digestive and bowel disorders, with diarrhoea and stomach pains, which continued for several days. On the eleventh day he developed a respiratory infection, with coughing, a sore throat and earache. For the next few days he was in discomfort from swellings in his neck and face. He was sleeping poorly and was unable to eat. On the eighteenth day he had a naso-gastric tube inserted to permit feeding. By the twentieth day following the commencement of chemotherapy he was generally feeling improved. His tube was removed, he was tolerating small amounts of food by mouth, he was able to leave his bed, walk to the toilet, and go out for a trip in town by wheelchair.

However, while Paul's apparent physical condition now appeared relatively stable, his mental condition began to give rise to concern. He began to display intermittent periods of confusion and agitation. These confusional episodes mostly occurred when Paul was trying to follow a routine sequence of motor acts (such as dressing or washing). Typically he would begin the process but then lose track of his intention and be unable to maintain and complete the activity. This breakdown of an otherwise automatic chain of motor sequences suggested the possibility of either a pharmacological or neurological disturbance, requiring further investigation.

Preliminary psychological assessment began to show the extent of his inability to execute many types of psychomotor activity. Information about Paul's pre-morbid intellectual and psychological state had showed no evidence of any unusual features. Now, however, assessment of his general cognitive abilities (Wechsler, 1974) showed a significant discrepancy between auditory-vocal and visual-motor functions. While he was still able to function at average levels for his age on verbal tasks,he was quite unable to cope even at the level of a 5-year-old child on most non-verbal tasks, displaying gross distortions of visuospatial abilities. Similarly, his ability to complete a pencil and paper task of copying a series of patterns (Bender, 1946) showed a level of confusion and a quality of errors frequently associated with cerebral dysfunction.

A more detailed neuropsychological examination (Christiansen, 1975) was therefore completed. This indicated the possibility of a lesion in the parieto-occipital area. Paul could not make simple judgements based on visuo-spatial information (he could no longer tell the time from an hour/minute hand clock, he could not follow a game of noughts and crosses). He experienced changes in his perception of external objects, with distortion of their size and shape (he reported seeing his dressing gown growing in size whilst hanging on the door), he could not judge distances (when reaching for a drink he might miss, he could not trust his judgement of the position of a chair beneath him when sitting down). In addition to these problems, Paul's already observed difficulty in maintaining and directing a sequence of actions suggested a possible further cerebral lesion. When given the task of copying a mixed sequence of visual patterns he would persevere with one pattern. He displayed motor echopraxia when asked to imitate a series of different motor actions, despite being able to repeat the original verbal instructions correctly. This tendency to revert to an initial stereotype uncontrolled by verbal regulation led to the break down of his plans of action, and to a loss of intention. These examples of confused behaviour and inability to maintain goal-directed behaviour suggested a frontal lobe defect.

The presence of lesions in the parieto-occipital and frontal lobes was confirmed by CT scan. It was subsequently discovered that these were three cerebral abscesses arising from aspergillosis, a fungal infection of his brain. Six weeks now after his admission to hospital, Paul underwent neurosurgery for aspiration of the abscesses and insertion of an Omaya reservoir for cerebral drainage. He was by now in remission but had only completed the induction phase of his chemotherapy. Further cytotoxic treatment was suspended, and he began intensive antibiotic therapy for treatment of his critical cerebral condition. After an early setback requiring further surgery, Paul slowly began to recover. By the ninth week from admission he was considered well enough to undergo the cranial irradiation phase of his original treatment protocol. However, because he had had such a traumatic experience as a result of induction chemotherapy it was decided not to proceed with the two phases of intensification. As a result, now 11 weeks on, he was discharged from hospital and returned home.

Recovery from aspergillosis is rare. There is little evidence, therefore, to guide us about neurological recovery in these cases. I had been monitoring Paul's psychological status throughout his hospitalization. An early repeat psychological assessment 1 week after his second operation already showed a modest improvement in some intellectual functions. Paul was now trying to use verbal strategies to overcome his visuoperceptual problems, by talking himself through tasks. He could, with some hesitation, work out the time by verbally labelling hours and minutes on the clock face. However, he was still vulnerable to loss of intention in completing a sequence of motor acts, but with the difference that he did not become as agitated as before. He was conscious of his difficulties and was prepared to use alternative strategies to overcome them.

Some 3 months after the initial identification of his neurological dysfunction, I saw Paul at his family home for a complete psychological reassessment. He now displayed an almost complete functional recovery of all neurological processes. He presented as mentally alert and provided some insights into his experiences when neurologically disabled. He recalled his initial attempts to copy a diamond shape "I could see what it was clearly enough, I knew it was a diamond. But I couldn't seem to get my hand to do it. I couldn't figure out which direction to draw the line". This problem of recognizing the total gestalt but not synthesizing the components operated in a different direction when he tried to tell the time. "I knew it was a clock, but I couldn't recognize the time. I knew the hour hand, the minute hand and the numbers. But I couldn't seem to match up both hands to their numbers. I could work out one of them, like the hours, but I couldn't then convert the numbers for the other hand to minutes. There seemed too much to have to work out all at the same time". In the familiar surroundings of his home, Paul was mostly coping adequately with routine activities. He did note that if he had too many things to do at once it was "like overloading my circuits. I have to be careful that I don't get flustered, otherwise I don't cope at all". That was how it had been in hospital when confusional episodes were noted. He described how, for example, he would begin to wash. He would put the plug in the sink and start to fill it up with water. Then he might forget what to do next, whether to reach for the soap, find a towel, take off his pyjama jacket, and meanwhile the sink would continue to fill with water and he would panic. In hospital he would often be rescued by a nurse, who would take over the operation and calm him down.

Eight months after his initial diagnosis, I saw Paul again at his home. He had now been back at his school for 2 months. While he now seemed entirely free of visuospatial disturbance, the more open-ended and distracting environment of school was exposing his residual vulnerability to loss of intention and self-direction. He noted that he needed to be more consciously vigilant than before in routine behaviour, otherwise he could be easily distracted. Following familiar routes around the school could sometimes lead to him arriving at the wrong lesson. "I sometimes have to keep telling myself where I'm meant to be going. If I start to day-dream I might find myself taking the wrong way." However Paul was active in trying to develop strategies to compensate. He was making regular use of his school diary to direct himself from lesson to lesson, and deliberately setting out his books on his desk to remind himself which ones he needed for each day. He noted "I still can have my off-days, and then I've got to be conscious of what I'm doing. It's like I have to get back into the swing of it, but sometimes it can be very difficult".

The active coping strategies that Paul was now adopting were, however, different from those he mostly used in hospital. "In hospital you just have to be patient. There's nothing you can do most of the time, and you've just got to accept it." However, in school he was expected to take more responsibility for what occurred, to be more active in that environment. The stressors that we had identified as bothering Paul most when he was in hospital were to do with pain and discomfort from treatment, frustration from hospitalization, and uncertainty and anxiety about his future. Stressful physical features were identified as feeling unwell, (aches and pains, nausea, lack of energy) and hurt of needles. Stressful psychological factors were occasioned by enforced inactivity (being restricted to bed, attached to a drip), anticipation of hurtful medical procedures, and uncertainty about the future. Paul used similar coping strategies for feeling unwell and enforced inactivity. These took the form of acceptance ("grin and bear it"), positive cognitions ("it can't last for ever", "it's all part of the treatment I need"), the use of distraction (having father read him humorous stories), and the use of avoidance ("I try and sleep as much as I can when I'm not feeling well"). He consciously attempted to use muscular relaxation and stimulus distraction when receiving injections, and was at least able to maintain a level of coping with, if not a level of mastery over, injections. Paul's anticipation of future painful medical procedures and anxiety about an uncertain future were met with denial, or at least avoidance. e.g. "I try to shut it all out . . . try not to think about it . . put it out of my mind and think of something else". There were also elements of regression to a state of greater dependency, by placing more reliance in the doctors and on his parents to take decisions on his behalf, to achieve a sort of vicarious confidence by trusting these adults to make the right judgements for him.

By using a range of coping behaviours that were mostly emotion-focused, or palliative strategies, Paul managed to limit the debilitating effects of hospital stress.

Back in school, however, he had to adopt more active, independent behaviours. Paul observed that he had to be more self-reliant, to do things for himself, to respond to several stimuli at once, but to actively maintain the focus of his concentration on the appropriate target. The recent social and neurological consequences of his illness and treatment may have now made this difficult for him to do. The coping strategies he had developed were mostly problem-focused. He was deliberately organizing his day, making plans for meeting the demands of school activities, thinking things out, so that mainly he was vigilant, active and personally responsible for his life now. At the same time he was aware of the need for emotion-focused responses, to stay relaxed and "keep calm under pressure" and to develop confidence by positive thinking ("I tell myself I can do it").

In both settings, hospital and school, Paul was able to make use of the mechanism of social support. In hospital that had been mostly at a level of delegating the work of worrying to his parents and responsibility for his physical well-being to the medical staff. In school it was a more interactive, shared process. When problems arose Paul would talk them over with his teachers or his parents. He was conscious of their support, and confident that he could rely on them to modify demands that taxed his abilities and to provide guidance to develop alternative strategies. While this paper is concerned with Paul's response to various stressors, we cannot make proper account of that without having regard to the response of his family. As I earlier observed, studies of stress and coping in children and young people must include the social dimension of, at least, their families whose role is often to provide a stress buffer. Nine months after his initial admission to hospital Paul's parents were able to observe that he had displayed much less emotional distress than they had anticipated at the outset. On the other hand they also recognized that they themselves had coped much worse than they had predicted. The emotional demands of their son's illness, hospitalization and treatment had been very stressful, and they had not always been able to call upon coping strategies adequate to those demands. While they had provided Paul with valuable psychological support, they themselves had found it difficult to avoid or resolve conflicts concerning their son's treatment.

The role demands of patient and pupil, or parent of patient and pupil, called for different responses. Paul's assumption of the patient role produced passivity and dependence. When he resumed the role of pupil he was able to shift back to a more interactive and self-directive mode of behaving. On the other hand the role of "parent of pupil" was one that

Paul's parents had played passively ("leave it up to school, they know best"). That was not a role they chose to assume, however, in the hospital where perhaps their hyper-vigilance led to tensions between parents and hospital staff.

The intention of this case study has been to describe the various physiological, psychological and social stresses that in various ways and at various times were acting upon one adolescent patient over a period of 9 months. Because of his recovery from a short-term neurological disorder he was able to provide some insight into his experience when perceptually disorientated, and to develop some compensatory strategies in attempting to overcome it. His experiences as a patient, and later again as a student, suggest that coping is not a fixed function, but rather depends on a flexible range of strategies whose appropriateness depends upon the circumstances. Folkman and Lazarus (1980) have attempted to categorize coping strategies broadly as being emotion-focused or problem focused. While I have suggested that in Paul's case his coping responses in hospital tended to be more emotion-focused and in school to be more problem-focused, the distinction in reality is less clear. If we considered processes that appear emotional ("how do I feel?"), cognitive ("what do I think?") or behavioural ("what do I do?") in Paul's response to stressors we may observe that they interact more than they separate. His anxiety about needles in hospital might provide an example. "How do I *feel* when I *think* about my next injection?" involves cognitive appraisal of an emotional response. "I *feel* like that when I *think* about injections, so I will try not to think about it" suggests an act of cognitive self-control to resolve the problem of experiencing upsetting emotions. "How will I *behave* when the needle goes in?" invites the use of cognitions to monitor and control behavioural responses. "I will relax my muscles, I will look at something else. I will get the nurse to talk with me while the doctor is inserting the needle." His strategies for managing the stresses at school were likewise a merging of cognitive, emotional and behavioural processes. "I am aware that when I think that I have too much homework to do I start to feel panic. I know that when I panic I cannot think efficiently . . . I will tell myself that I can do it. I will relax, keep calm. I will ask my teacher for help if I need it." Dealing with a stressful problem involves a disturbing emotional response: dealing with a disturbing emotion involves a problem-solving activity.

Paul's adaptive responses to stressful events served to limit their effects. He seemed successful in resisting the debilitating effects of various stressors so that he was able to tolerate his hospitalization and make a good readjustment to school. In this the social support of his parents, teachers and hospital staff became part of his own coping system. Coping strategies were determined by situational demands, which predicted the role behaviour, and each made use of a span of responses in which so-called cognitive, emotional and behavioural features were interwined.

REFERENCES

Bender, L. (1946) *Visual Motor Gestalt Test.*American Orthopsychiatric Association.
Christiansen, A. (1975) *Luria's Neuropsychological Investigation.*Spectrum, New York.
Folkman, S. and Lazarus, R. S. (1980) An analysis of coping in a middle-aged community sample. *J. Health Soc. Behav.* **21,** 219–239
Garmezy, N. and Rutter, M. (Eds) (1983) *Stress, Coping and Development in Children* McGraw-Hill. New York.
Wechsler, D. (1974) *Wechsler Intelligence Scale for Children—Revised.* Psychological Corporation. New York.

The Problems of a Child's Return to School

ANNE CHARLTON

ABSTRACT

Now that the cure rate for children's cancers has risen so sharply in recent years, more and more children are returning to school either during or after treatment. It is generally agreed that it is best to get back to normal life as soon as possible. But this situation is comparatively new and presents its own problems.

Prior to a large scale study, a small pilot study was carried out. This study funded by the Cancer Research Campaign looked at the problems experienced by some young former cancer patients, their teachers and families.

The results are based on "in-depth" interviews with the parents and teachers of 16 children who had been off treatment for 2 or more years and had therefore returned to school on a normal basis.

Five important factors emerged clearly:

1. Children whose treatment was right at the start of their schooling had severe integration problems.
2. Children at secondary school had special anxieties about specific academic subjects they needed for future qualifications.
3. Prostheses present many and varied problems.
4. Teasing by other children was a frequent problem.
5. Siblings often developed problems.

Most teachers and parents would have welcomed advice and or help with these problems and it is hoped that, when the larger scale Cancer Research Campaign-funded study has clarified the finer points, some system for helping will be devised.

Not so many years ago the prognosis of most childhood cancers was so poor that returning to normal school life after treatment was rarely possible. Even in the few cases where it was feasible, parents, teachers and doctors were often opposed to the child's being "forced" to work when so little life might be left to him.

Now the situation has completely changed. Many childhood cancers now have a very good prognosis and there is no doubt that most people involved in the child's care and treatment — perhaps most of all the child him- or herself — feel that a prompt return to the normal routine of school life can be of great benefit to the child.

Clearly this return to school could present problems. Any absence, no matter how short and for whatever reasons, can lead to difficulties, but long or repeated absences during which the child has undergone aggressive treatment *could* present a situation fraught with problems.

Our aim, must if it is all possible, be to prevent these problems from

PO—C

21

arising, or if they are inevitable, to forestall and alleviate them as far as possible. But in order to do this, we need to know what difficulties are likely to be encountered and what causes them. A great deal of research has been carried out on this subject in the United States of America (Green, 1975; Lansky *et al.*, 1975; Sachs, 1980; Cairns *et al.*, 1982; Spinetta, 1982; Ross and Scarvalone, 1982; Henning and Fritz, 1983; Stehbens *et al.*, 1983) but very little has been done in this country. Since the education system, the medical system, and the people are different in America from those of the U.K., we cannot automatically transfer their findings and solutions to our own situation.

The project described in this paper was therefore developed by two consultants, Dr Pat Morris-Jones and Dr Dorothy Pearson, and myself in order to identify the problems and to provide some solutions. At present we have completed the pilot study and its findings will be used in the planning of a large scale study.

SAMPLE AND METHODS

The sample consisted of the parents and teachers of 20 children who had been treated for solid tumours and had been off treatment for 2 years. Solid tumour patients were selected because most of the work which has already been carried out in this country has concentrated on leukaemia patients. Sixteen of the original sample participated in the study.

The types of tumour included two osteosarcomas, two Ewing's sarcomas, three brain tumours, a teratoma of the ovary, a rhabdomyosarcoma of the orbit, a thalamic glioma, a spinal tumour, a chondrosarcoma, a lymphoma of the appendix, a dysgerminoma, a squamous epithelial carcinoma of an alveolus, and a spinal tumour.

The study consisted of in-depth interviews with the parents and teachers. Permission was first obtained from the appropriate Ethical Committees, and the General Practitioner for each patient was informed and asked to let us know any contra-indications he knew of for interviewing that particular family.

The interviews with parents were carried out in the child's home or at the outpatients' clinic according to the parents' preferences. The teachers' interviews were carried out in the schools. Both parents and teachers were given the option of sending in the questionnaire by post and a few did so.

The respondents were assured of confidentiality and were told that if they preferred not to answer any question or if they wished the interview to stop, their decision would be final.

RESULTS

Because this was a pilot study we wanted to look at as many aspects as possible. In a brief paper it is not feasible to go through all the findings in detail, but the main points are summarized.

(a) Practical aspects of the return to school

Most of the parents were advised by the paediatric oncologist that their child was fit to return to school and most of the parents (63%) and the children themselves (88%) felt that it was time for this transition to take place. Two of the children did not want to return, due to fear or apathy, but others were keen to get back to their friends, or make up their lost work, and one or two were just bored at home. Almost all the parents commented on the relief of "getting back to normal" which was created by the child's return to school.

Only one of the teachers, however, claimed to have received any information or advice about the child's return other than from the parents or from the pupil him or herself. Six of the schools did not know what treatment the child had received, and it was almost always the parents who informed the school of special problems which might arise. Ten of the schools said that nobody had contacted them to discuss any problems which might be expected and almost all said they would have welcomed some information and advice on this. In fact all schools are contacted as a matter of course, but it appears that the information does not always reach the right teachers.

Thirteen of the schools said that they had been given no information as to where advice and help could be sought if difficulties arose, but most of them said they would have liked to have contact with someone who could provide re-assurance.

(b) The best and worst things about returning to school

The five best things from the children's point of view were:
    being back with their friends (38%);
    getting back to normal (19%);
    getting out of the house, being occupied and getting a broader outlook (19%);
    getting back into the school system (13%); and
    picking up on missed work and not getting too far behind (6%).
The worst things for the children were mainly *worries:*
    about loss of hair (38%) or physical problems (13%);
    about not being able to catch up on work (13%)
    about how their friends would react to them (13%);
    about their small size (6%); and
    about being put in a low academic group and wanting to go up (6%).
The best things for *parents* were almost always the return to normality, but seeing the child happy, reunited with his or her friends and not getting too far behind with work were all important elements too.
As with the children, the worst things for parents were *worries;*

that he or she might not be able to cope with school life (31%);
about other children teasing or possible rejection by friends (31%);
about the possibility of physical injuries (19%);
about loss of hair (19%); and
about loss of so much school-work (6%).
Were these worries, in fact, justified? In some cases they were.

(c) Physical problems

Only one teacher gave a completely unqualified "no" when asked if the child had any physical problems, although only half the parents said their child had any. The school is probably far more likely than the home situation to put the child in a position where physical difficulties become apparent. The teachers frequently mentioned specific problems with school activities and expressed the need for help or advice. Some of the problems were as follows:

tiredness, and loss of interest (31%);
problems with the prosthesis (in this case, the leg) (13%);
difficulties in moving around the school (13%);
the wig in PE lessons (6%);
the need for fluids, eye drops, etc. during lessons (6%); and
the problems of coping with practical subjects which require the use of the arm or other affected limb (6%).

The parents also usually mentioned tiredness (31%) and the frustration of the child at his or her inadequacy in the sports, play or other activities which had been important to him or her before the illness (50%).

Physical education could have presented problems, but eleven of the teachers said it had not, usually because the parents had defined clear limits for the child. Some schools (31%) arranged alternative activities for the child during PE lessons, but for those who were specially keen on particular sports, efforts were made to let them participate in so far as they could. Many of the teachers (63%) were extremely anxious as to the extent of participation which was advisable, and they sometimes felt that they erred on the side of caution. Some medical guidelines would have been appreciated in almost all cases.

One girl was given very special protection and help by her school. She was allowed to go to eat her sandwiches in the room for handicapped pupils, which had special facilities and ladies to take care of its occupants. She rejected this in favour of the girls' toilets. It is possible for schools to show a tendency to overwhelm the returning pupils with kindness and make them feel isolated and in the "sick role" when in fact they are feeling well, hope they are recovered, and want to get back to normal with their own class group.

Prostheses sometimes presented special problems to the five children who had them. In the first instance they were always a disappointment, having been eagerly awaited by the child as the means to become normal and be able to do everything again. Once the limitations had been accepted, further problems arose. Limb supply in the North of England appears to be slow and sometimes a limb was too small by the time it arrived for fitting. This meant a day or half a day off school, with no new limb at the end of it. One particular girl had tremendous problems with her artificial leg which frequently fell to pieces and had to be repaired in the Science laboratory at school. The metal parts tore her skirt, and the limb frequently let her down, so much so that she often preferred to take it off rather than cope with it.

It is hoped that the methods of treatment recently introduced will largely eliminate the need for artificial limbs of this kind for children, but there still appears to be a need for a considerable improvement in limb supply and manufacture for those young people for whom there is no alternative.

(d) Academic work and achievement

The parents were, on the whole, rather concerned about their children's missed work. The big problem with the secondary school children was missing mathematics. No other specific problem was mentioned. The youngest primary school children also seemed to have great difficulty in catching up. To hazard a guess as to the reasons for these problems, both mathematics and the first infant school stages need definite teaching of basic principles. A lot of other subjects and junior school work relies on reading and can be easily learned by private study. The reception class at infants' school also covers that important step from being a "baby" to being a schoolchild. To miss this step when contemporaries are taking it can be a major problem.

There was a general tendency among the children to feel "left behind". Schoolfriends often helped by taking work round to the child, but of course, the usefulness of this depends on the academic level of the helpful friend. About half of the children were extremely hard on themselves and achieved results every bit as good as if they had not been ill.

Nine of the schools sent work whilst the child was absent from school. Two children had no long absences due to their treatment being in the summer holiday. In another case the teacher visited the child in the evenings to teach her class work. Six of the pupils who were sent work from school did it.

None had a home tutor and only four parents would have wanted them to have one. The teachers' opinions on home tutors varied widely. Some were definitely against having them and others were equally strongly in favour. The point which the teachers stressed most was the vital importance of home tutors and hospital teachers going to the school before planning the lessons and teaching *exactly* what the child's own class is doing in *exactly* the same way.

At least one of the children had become very lazy due to her absence. Her teacher said "She was very lazy. She took advantage and had difficulty settling back. Her work went off and she needed shouting at. It is difficult for people to know that she can be treated normally." This last sentence summed up a lot of worries which the teachers had about the child's return. How far should he or she be pushed or punished? One teacher said "People didn't expect as much. Perhaps they should. They didn't pressure him to work." Most of these children (69%) had very definite careers in view: e.g. a fashion designer, a doctor, a computer technician, work with animals or children, a career in the Army or Navy. To help them achieve their aims they need to achieve certain academic goals. One said her career would be particularly important if she could not have children. If they want it enough they do not mind being pushed. It also helps them to return to being a normal member of the class. Such observations as "She caught up in the first 12 months. She got A in all subjects" were gratifying to the child, teacher and parents.

(e) Psychological problems

Nine of the teachers reported that the child had no problems of this kind, and some were surprised that they did not. The others showed various difficulties, one became quieter, two more belligerent or demanding. One wanted attention all the time in class, two regressed to thumb-sucking. Two became very gloomy and tearful from time to time. One child had more severe disturbance which manifested itself in many ways, but was mainly based on complete isolation from her peers.

(f) Classmates

Cancer is so surrounded by fear, mystery and misconceptions, how would the classmates react? They ranged from being overprotective to being completely unconcerned. There were a few negative reactions. One mother said "His classmates were distant. He didn't look the same lad and they didn't recognize him. It was a big physical change and they were frightened to go near him." Most negative reactions occurred in children in other classes rather than those in the child's own class. They called names such as "cancer boy", "Quasimodo" and "bald head". When the children had all been prepared by their teacher for the return they were usually better.

Most, but not all, the classes kept in touch with tapes, letters, cards, presents and visits whilst the child was away. Before the return they asked many questions such as

"What's a tumour?"

"Is a tumour the same as cancer?"

"How did they get inside her head?"

"What's an artificial leg like?"

Five of the teachers said they would have liked some help in dealing with these questions.

(g) Siblings

Siblings of a sick child can need special attention both in and out of school. All these children had siblings. Their reactions appeared to fall largely into the following categories:

worry;

puzzlement e.g. "They found it very difficult to understand. She was never really ill. They thought she was skiving off school.";

jealousy;

fear "don't bring her home. I don't want to see her again.";

support for parents; and

protectiveness to the sick child.

Some siblings apparently showed no adverse reactions, but some parents suspected that they were just concealing their concern.

"Her younger brother lay awake at night and was probably more worried than he knew".

Others reacted very badly, throwing tantrums in school, withdrawing into themselves and in one or two cases showing fairly severe psychological problems.

CONCLUSION

On the whole, these children of junior school age appeared to have the least problems in returning to school. There could be two main reasons for this.

1. They are at a stage when illnesses of all kinds are frequent among children. To be away with cancer is given no more emphasis among the children than to be away with measles or mumps. As one mother said of her son's classmates

   "All seemed to have had bigger operations and had bigger scars to show".

2. Much of the learning at this stage is either consolidation or the acquisition of new information which can be attained by reading.

What seems to help the child's return is that he or she should have:

independence;
interests and aims;
· school support;
frankness; and
better artificial limbs supplied more easily.

Parents and teachers felt that they needed more information on "do's and don'ts". The teachers especially would have welcomed not only some written information for ready reference, but also a "hotline" to a person with specific medical knowledge, about this particular child, who could help or advise in emergency.

Many of the teachers and parents felt that the image of cancer in the minds of the general public plays a tremendous part in causing problems for the returning child. More realistic knowledge of the cancers could help very greatly.

The ambivalent feeling with which parents entrust their child back to the care of the school was expressed by this mother who, when asked if anything else could have been done to make her son's return easier for her, said "No. Only if I could have gone with him to hold his hand."

We must never lose sight of the fact that the child, no matter how sick he has been, or even still is, has his or her place in the world, his or her hopes and fears and usually a goal, no matter how impractical this may appear. We must all help him or her to achieve it. Hopes do not automatically vanish with illness.

ACKNOWLEDGEMENT

Printed with permission as a shorter report on the study described in the paper published in *Social Science and Medicine* Vol. 22, pages 1337 — 1346, 1986 A. Charlton, D. Pearson and P. Morris-Jones, Children's return to school after treatment for solid tumours. The author's most grateful thanks are due to the Cancer Research Campaign for financing this research and to all the parents and teachers who helped us so much.

REFERENCES

Cairns, N. U., Klopovich, P., Hearne, E. and Lansky, S. B. (1982) School attendance of children with cancer. *J. Sch. H.* March, 152—155.
Green, P. (1975) The child with leukaemia in the classroom. *Am J. Nurs.* **75**, 86—87,
Henning, J. and Fritz, G. K. (1983) School re-entry in childhood cancer. *Psychosomatics* **23**, 261—269.
Lansky, S. B., Lowman, J. T., Vats, T. S. and Gyulay, J. E. (1975) School phobia in children with malignant neoplasma. *Am. J. Dis. Child.* **129**, 42—46.
Ross, J. W. and Scarvalone, S. A. (1982) Facilitating the paediatric cancer patient's return to school. *Soc. Work* **27**, 256—261.
Sachs, M. B. (1980) Helping the child with cancer to go back to school. *J. Sch. Health.* 328—331.
Spinetta, J. J. (1982) Behavioral and psychological research in childhood cancer. An overview. *Cancer 50 Suppl.* **50**, 1934—1945.
Stehbens, J. A., Kisker, C. T. and Wilson, B. K. (1983) School behavior and attendance during the first year of treatment for childhood cancer. *Psychol. Sch.* **20**, 223—228.

PART TWO

Adult Cancers

A. Epidemiology

Cancer Mortality and Widow(er)hood in the Office of Population Censuses and Surveys: Longitudinal Study*

D. R. JONES

ABSTRACT

Many studies have suggested that following the experience of "stressful" life events the risks of myocardial infarction, accidents and perhaps other diseases including cancer are elevated. In the OPCS Longitudinal Study (LS) routinely collected data on deaths, and deaths of a spouse occurring in a 1% sample of the population of England and Wales in the period 1971—1981 are linked together and with 1971 census records of sample members. The timing and patterns of death following the potentially very stressful event of conjugal bereavement may thus be analysed.

Overall the mortality in widowers, but not widows, was about 10% in excess of that in all members of the LS sample for most major causes of death groups. As in many earlier studies, some increases in death rates shortly after widow(er)hood are observed. Unusually, for deaths from all causes these increases are more marked in widows than in widowers, with, for example, a twofold increase in mortality from all causes in the first month after widowhood. However, no peak of post-bereavement mortality from malignant diseases is clearly established in either sex.

The observed patterns, although consistent with an early effect of a stressful life event, do not strongly suggest that stress following bereavement leads to an excess of cancer mortality. The limited follow-up of the study cohort since widowhood must, however, be kept in mind.

Although there is a long history of reported associations between "stress" and cancer with many references to the importance of the loss of a relationship or of a near relative (e.g. Snow, 1893; Evans, 1926; Le Shan, 1966), early studies were based mainly on potentially biased case reports. As Ramirez (1987) comments, many "life event" studies in this field suffer from familiar problems of this methodology, including retrospective ascertainment of the life events, incomplete and possibly inappropriately weighted life event scales, no measures of contextual meaning of the life events, inadequate (or even absent) control groups and small sample sizes, exacerbated in this context by psychosocial adjuncts of the diagnosis of cancer. Although some positive associations between loss events and cancer have been reported [for example, by Horne and Picard (1980) and Cooper et al., (1986)], negative results [such as those of Greer & Morris (1975), Priestman et al. (1985), Ewertz (1986)] predominate. In view of the methodological limitations of many of the studies no firm overall conclusion is, however, yet clear.

This caution is further prompted by the lack of clear identification of mechanisms of carcinogenesis following "stress" (Rosch, 1984) although neuroendocrinological and immunological pathways seem likely (Pettingale, 1985). Of particular relevance here is the direct evidence of depressed lymphocyte levels following bereavement (Schleifer et al., 1983).

Loss of a spouse is potentially among the most stressful of life events (Holmes and Rahe, 1967) but the response of the bereaved spouse to the loss of his/her partner is likely to depend on many factors, some of them specific to the bereaved person and his/her circumstances at the time of bereavement rather than to the nature of the loss event (Parkes, 1986; Craig and Brown, 1984).

This paper describes the results obtained in the course of a large prospective study (Fox and Goldblatt, 1982) based on linkage of data from the 1971 Census with subsequent routinely-collected data on mortality.

An earlier study of cancer registration and death rates following widow(er)hood from the same data source has already been described elsewhere (Jones et al., 1984). There was very little evidence of an increase in cancer registration rates following widow(er)hood, and only a weak suggestion of increased death rates, as a result of reduced survival from incidence of cancer to death in the widow(er)ed. Overall, the earlier study provides little positive evidence for a link between bereavement and cancer. Indeed, it quite strongly suggests that a large excess of cancer registrations of death will not be seen shortly after widow(er)hood. More details of the further results described here and a brief review of the results of previous studies of post-bereavement mortality are given elsewhere (Jones and Goldblatt, 1986).

Mechanisms other than stress resulting from bereavement may lead to post-bereavement mortality excess (Jacobs and Ostfeld, 1979; Susser, 1981). Possible alternative mechanisms include: (i) homogamy — a tendency of spouses to have similar physical and mental characteristics (Ciocco, 1940; Jones and Goldblatt, 1987), (ii) common marital environment, including the sharing of many aspects of life style, (iii) simultaneous death of husband and wife, especially in a single accident or violent incident (when the younger partner is conventionally regarded as having been widow(er)ed), (iv) loss of spousal support (Kaplan et al., 1977) in respect of nursing or other care, a reduction in motivation, a less adequate diet, increased poverty, or changes in social networks and contacts, and (v) postponement of death during illness of the spouse, especially where one spouse is caring for the other spouse during terminal illness. All of these possible alternative explanations should be kept in mind as we examine the results from the present study.

SUBJECTS AND METHODS

The Office of Population Censuses and Surveys (OPCS) Longitudinal Study (LS) was initiated on the basis of a 1% sample of individuals enumerated in England and Wales in the 1971 Census. For this initial sample, 1971 Census records have been linked to subsequent routinely collected information about these individuals. These event data are obtained from other routine OPCS data systems such as the birth, death and cancer registration systems. Limited data on the family and household of sample members are included in the study in several ways, two of which are relevant here. First, information from the death record of a spouse of a sample member, and second, census data relating to other members of any household which included an LS member are linked with the information about the sample member. The subsequent mortality patterns of sample members whose spouses died in the period between the 1971 and 1981 Censuses are the main focus of interest in the present study. Approximately 85% of widow(er)hoods in the LS sample have been fully linked into the study; almost 100% of subsequent mortality of the widow(er)s is, however, recorded. The mean length of post-bereavement follow-up in the results presented here was 4.5 years for widows and 4.0 years for widowers.

Several different analyses using these LS data are reported here. In all the analyses, the numbers of deaths expected in the group studied were calculated (see Fox and Goldblatt, 1982) by a standard procedure (Berry, 1983). Deaths are categorized by underlying causes, coded according to the Eighth Revision of International Classification of Diseases (World Health Organization, 1969). Approximate 95% confidence limits calculated by the method of Vandenbroucke (1982) for the ratio of observed to expected deaths are given for most table entries.

Two distinct types of standard group have been used in highlighting different issues in these analyses. In some of the analyses the standard groups comprise all LS sample members of the same sex as the group studied, irrespective of whether or not they had suffered bereavement. To control for year of bereavement and survival since bereavement, standard group rates were calculated from a simulated, randomly-timed event in each year for each LS member. In the remaining analyses all widows or widowers in the LS form the standard group with which sub-groups of widows or widowers are compared, and in these analyses

TABLE 1. MORTALITY IN 1971—1981 FOLLOWING WIDOW(ER)HOOD EARLIER IN THE PERIOD 1971—1981, BY CAUSE AND SEX

	Sex	
Cause of death of widow(er)	Females (widows)	Males (widowers)
All causes	2202 (2132.3)	1939 (1734.7)
	1.03 (0.99–1.08)	1.12 (1.07–1.17)
All malignant neoplasms	413 (418.3)	383 (357.2)
(ICD: 140-209)	0.99 (0.89–1.09)	1.07 (0.97–1.18)
Disease of the circulatory system	1206 (1167.2)	1013 (899.8)
(ICD: 390-458)	1.03 (0.97–1.09)	1.13 (1.06–1.20)
Disease of the respiratory system	288 (293.3)	348 (326.8)
(ICD: 460-519)	0.98 (0.87–1.10)	1.06 (0.95–1.18)
Accidents, poisonings and violence	73 (47.1)	49 (29.6)
(ICD: 800-999)	1.55 (1.21–1.93)	1.66 (1.22–2.16)

Table entries: observed (expected*) deaths; ratio observed/expected (approx. 95% confidence interval for ratio).
*Based on age and sex-specific death rates in the whole LS sample in 1971-1981.

survival was measured from date of bereavement in both standard and studied groups.

RESULTS

Of the 133,007 married men in the LS sample at the 1971 Census 7,060 suffered widow(er)hood before the end of 1981; in the same period 14,900 of the 131,277 married women in the sample were widowed. In this paper deaths in 1971–1981 *following* widow(er)hood in 1971–1981 amongst the complete cohorts of married men and women enumerated at the 1971 Census are analysed.

Table 1 shows observed and expected mortality in widows and widowers, allowing comparison of observed death rates in these groups with the rates in age and sex-matched groups in which marital status is unrestricted. Deaths of widows and widowers occurring on the *same* day as the death of their spouses are omitted from this table. The data for widows provide little evidence of an excess of mortality from any major group of underlying cause, compared to that in the whole female population, with the obvious exception of death from accidents, poisonings or violent causes where an approximate 50% excess can be seen. In the widowers, excesses of around 10% are seen in all of the major disease groups except for accidents, poisonings and violence in which the excess is again much larger. These excess mortality rates in widow(er)s are generally somewhat less marked than those seen in cross-sectional studies (Registrar General, 1971).

The variation of excess mortality with age is shown in Table 2 to be different in widows and widowers; in widows the excess from all causes of death is marked only below age 65 whereas the excess is apparent at

TABLE 2. MORTALITY IN 1971—1981 FOLLOWING WIDOW(ER)HOOD EARLIER IN THE PERIOD BY CAUSE AND AGE GROUP

Age group	All causes of death		Deaths from malignant neoplasms	
	Widows	Widowers	Widows	Widowers
≤64	395 (348.9)	285 (243.1)	134 (128.2)	74 (73.6)
	1.13 (1.02-1.25)	1.17 (1.04-1.32)	1.05 (0.87-1.23)	1.01 (0.79-1.25)
65-74	821 (830.2)	743 (6661.5)	168 (177.6)	187 (157.1)
	0.99 (0.92-1.06)	1.12 (1.04-1.21)	0.95 (0.81-1.10)	1.19 (1.02-1.37)
75 +	986 (953.2)	911 (830.2)	111 (112.5)	122 (126.6)
	1.03 (0.97-1.10)	1.10 (1.03-1.17)	0.99 (0.81-1.18)	0.96 (0.80-1.15)
All ages	2202 (2132.3)	1939 (1734.7)	413 (418.3)	383 (357.2)
	1.30 (0.99-1.08)	1.12 (1.07-1.17)	0.99 (0.89-1.09)	1.07 (0.97-1.19)

Table entries: observed (expected*) deaths; ratio observed/expected (approx 95% confidence interval for this ratio)
*Based on age and sex-specific death rates in the whole LS sample.

all ages in widowers. For deaths from cancer clear variations with age group are absent; in widowers an excess can be discerned only in the 65–74 age group. The patterns of mortality in Tables 1 and 2 do not obviously support a hypothesis based on stress of bereavement leading to an excess of post-bereavement mortality from cancer, although the limited period of follow up in this study may weaken its power to detect raised mortality following a relatively long latent period.

Time since bereavement

The pattern of death in widows and widowers by the length of time between the event of bereavement which begins the widow(er)hood and the death of the widow(er) which terminates it in part helps to distinguish the effect of *being* a widow(er) from the effects of *becoming* a widow(er). Tables 3 and 4 present the basic results of the present study relevant to this issue. The mortality of widows from all causes in the month following their bereavement is seen to be greatly in excess of the expected figure in Table 3. Thereafter, the point estimate of the ratio of observed to expected deaths (effectively a standardized mortality ratio) declines steadily. The early excess for circulatory disease deaths is also clear, but that for accidents, poisoning and violence even more remarkable, and mortality from these causes apparently continues to be in excess of the expected figure for some time after bereavement. In contrast, the pattern of excess mortality from malignant diseases is again entirely unremarkable.

In Table 4 the excess of deaths in widowers in the month following their bereavement is seen to be less marked than that in widows. Thereafter, the point estimates again decline, although apparently not so rapidly as in the widows. Thus one interpretation of these results is that the excess mortality following bereavement is sharply clustered immediately

TABLE 3. MORTALITY IN 1971—1981 BY INTERVAL SINCE WIDOWHOOD BY CAUSE OF DEATH: FEMALES

Cause of death of widow	Interval in Days Since Widowhood				
	0	1–30	31–90	91–183	184 +
All causes	10	64 (32) 2.00 (1.53–2.53)	92 (65.9) 1.40 (1.12–1.70)	106 (102.3) 1.04 (0.84–1.25)	1940 (1932.1) 1.00 (0.96–1.05)
Malignant neoplasms (ICD: 140-209)	1	9 (7.1) 1.27 (0.56–2.25)	15 (14.2) 1.06 (0.58–1.67)	17 (21.2) 0.80 (0.46–1.24)	362 (375.8) 0.96 (0.86–1.07)
Diseases of the circulatory system (ICD: 390-458)	6	29 (16.9) 1.72 (1.14–2.40)	46 (35.3) 1.30 (0.95–1.72)	56 (56.4) 0.99 (0.75–1.28)	1075 (1058.6) 1.02 (0.95–1.08)
Accidents, poisoning and violence (ICD: 800-999)	2	7 (0.7) 10.00 (3.87–18.99)	5 (1.6) 3.13 (0.95–6.55)	5 (2.4) 2.08 (0.64–4.36)	56 (46.8) 1.20 (0.90–1.54)

Table entries: Observed (expected*) deaths; ratio observed/expected (approximate 95% confidence intervals for ratio)
*Based on age and survival-period-specific death rates 1971–1981 in all females in the LS sample.

following bereavement in the widows but is more dispersed over the following period in the widowers. The pattern of cause specific mortality broadly reflects that for all causes except that from accidents, poisonings and violence which again shows an early peak with generally raised values. The most interesting feature of mortality from cancer is the weak suggestion that such excesses as do occur are to be seen 6 months or more after bereavement. This could be taken as weak evidence in support of stress of bereavement causing excess mortality from cancer, with a relatively long interval between the start of widowerhood and the death from cancer of the widower.

A breakdown of the results presented for mortality from cancer of all sites to site specific mortality is again limited by the size of the study sample. In widows, the pattern of mortality from cancer of the breast (82 deaths overall) closely follows the results presented for all sites combined. Much the same is true of mortality from cancer of the lung in the widowers (147 deaths) although there is the weakest of suggestions of a longer delay before the peak of mortality is reached.

Causes of death in spouse pairs

Tables 5 and 6 explore the relationships between the cause of death of widow(er)s and cause of death of their spouses. Ciocco (1940) suggested that, if hypotheses based on homogamy or the shared marital environment were to have a role to play in the observed patterns of postwidow(er)hood mortality, cause of death would be alike in marital pairs more often than expected on the basis of chance. However, the

TABLE 4. MORTALITY IN 1971–1981 BY INTERVAL SINCE WIDOWERHOOD BY CAUSE OF DEATH: MALES

Cause of death of widower	0	1–30	31–90	91–183	184 +
			Interval in Days Since Widowerhood		
All causes	8	50 (33.4) 1.50 (1.10–1.95)	83 (66.4) 1.25 (0.99–1.54)	117 (97.7) 1.20 (0.99–1.43)	1689 (1537.2) 1.10 (1.06–1.15)
Malignant neoplasms (ICD: 140-209)	1	7 (6.8) 1.03 (0.40–1.95)	10 (13.8) 0.72 (0.34–1.26)	19 (20.9) 0.91 (0.54–1.37)	347 (315.7) 1.10 (0.98–1.22)
Diseases of the circulatory system (ICD: 390-458)	2	21 (17.0) 1.24 (0.75–1.83)	42 (35.0) 1.20 (0.86–1.60)	68 (50.0) 1.36 (1.05–1.71)	882 (797.8) 1.11 (1.03–1.18)
Accidents, poisonings and violence (ICD: 800-999)	3	6 (0.6) 10.00 (3.50–19.83)	2 (1.0) 2.00 (0.17–5.83)	4 (1.8) 2.22 (0.56–5.00)	37 (26.1) 1.42 (0.99–1.92)

Table entries: Observed (expected*) deaths; ratio observed/expected (approximate 95% confidence intervals for ratio)
*Based on age and survival-period-specific death rates 1971–1981 in all males in the LS sample.

TABLE 5. CONCORDANCE IN CAUSE OF DEATH IN 1971-1981 OF WIDOW(ER)S AND THEIR SPOUSES

Cause of death of both widow(er) and spouse	Widowers	Widows
Malignant neoplasms	106 (107.9) 0.98 (0.80–1.18)	109 (103.9) 1.05 (0.86–1.26)
Circulatory system diseases	550 (537.8) 1.02 (0.94–1.11)	640 (634.1) 1.01 (0.93–1.09)
Respiratory system diseases	40 (35.6) 1.12 (0.80–1.51)	54 (50.7) 1.07 (0.79–1.37)
Accidents, poisonings or violence	4 (1.5) 2.67 (0.67–6.00)	3 (1.2) 2.50 (0.45–6.22)
All causes	718 (697.2) 1.03 (0.95–1.11)	820 (804.9) 1.02 (0.95–1.09)

Table entries: observed (expected*) deaths; ratio observed/expected (approx. 95% confidence interval)
*Based on age, sex and survival-period-specific cancer death rates in all widow(er)s in 1971-1981 in the LS.

results in Table 5 confirm that observed and expected values are very close, including those for deaths from cancer. In contrast, Parkes et al. (1969) report an excess of 24% of observed over expected deaths overall. The present results thus provide no support for the alternative hypothesis of homogamy or common marital environment as explanations of excess of postbereavement mortality, particularly in respect of cancer deaths.

The distributions of causes of death of the spouses of widow(er)s who subsequently died of cancer is generally close to that expected, but further examination of the time to death (from all causes) in widows according to the predictability of their husband's death is of interest as

TABLE 6. ALL-CAUSE MORTALITY OF WIDOWS IN 1971–1981 BY SELECTED CAUSES OF HUSBAND'S DEATH
AND SURVIVAL PERIOD

Survival period (months) from husband's death	Husband died of:	
	Lung cancer	Accident or violence
Day 0	1	2
0 –	7 (4.9) 1.43 (0.55–2.71)	6 (0.7) 8.57 (3.00–17.0)
2 –	2 (7.0) 0.29 (0.02–0.83)	4 (1.5) 2.67 (0.67–6.00)
4 –	25 (24.3) 1.03 (0.66–1.48)	5 (3.1) 1.61 (0.49–3.38)
12 +	153 (158.4) 0.97 (0.82–1.13)	22 (18.7) 1.18 (0.73–1.73)
All (except day 0)	187 (194.6) 0.96 (0.82–1.11)	37 (23.9) 1.55 (1.08–2.10)

Table entries: observed (expected) deaths; ratio observed/expected (approx. 95% confidence interval for ratio)
*Based on age, sex and survival-period-specific cancer death rates in all widow(er)s in 1971–1981 in the LS.

the results in Table 6 show. Widows whose husbands' deaths, of accidental or violent causes, were largely unpredictable exhibit a much larger excess of postbereavement mortality than those whose husbands died of a "predictable" cause, lung cancer, in which a considerable period of terminal illness is likely. Both subgroups suffer a peak of mortality immediately following bereavement, but that in the subgroup whose husbands died of accidents or violence is quite remarkable. Although this suggests that the "broken heart" syndrome may be valid, it is in fact *not* the case that deaths due to ischaemic heart disease feature unduly in this excess (Jones, 1987). More detailed analyses of patterns of death in spouse pairs in the Longitudinal Study are available elsewhere (Jones and Goldblatt, 1987).

DISCUSSION

In summary, this paper aims to describe some of the main features of the pattern and magnitude of mortality, principally from cancer, following widow(er)hood in a large prospective study. Cancer mortality following widow(er)hood is little, if at all, in excess of that in all LS members. A peak of all cause mortality lasting for about 6 months after bereavement is seen in widows; in widowers the excess appears to be less sharp but visible over a more extended period. No such clear picture emerges for deaths from cancer, although the results in widowers offer weak support for an excess following a considerable "latent" period.

Further analyses to investigate and take account of other socio-demographic variables, such as measures of socio-economic status and other variables which may have an influence on the outcome of bereavement, are necessary and have to some extent been reported elsewhere (Jones and Goldblatt, 1986). Variations of post-bereavement mortality with household structure offer only limited confirmation of the patterns expected if children (and others) in a household provide support following bereavement and so reduce the risk of mortality in the surviving spouse. As the study of concordance of causes of death in husband and wife pairs shows, homogamy or common marital environment also appears to have a very limited role in explaining the excess.

The study clearly has major limitations; its size is insufficient at least as far as the younger widow(er)s are concerned, the range of socio-demographic data collected in the census is restricted, and key psychometric variables are not measured at all. Perhaps most crucially, the length of follow-up after widowerhood is in this analysis rather limited for unequivocal inferences to be drawn about the mortality from a disease with a potentially long latent interval. Further problems may arise from the measurement of variables at the 1971 census, before widow(er)hood has occurred. Nonetheless, the study does not suffer from the major size and selectivity defects of several previous studies in this field, since it is based on a representative prospective sample with well matched controls, and an independently defined exit event.

The findings may help to identify the size and nature of mortality following bereavement and hence to specify appropriate and efficient bereavement counselling and other services. It is, for example, important in this regard to distinguish as far as possible between the stress and loss of support explanations of post bereavement mortality excesses. Although the stress of bereavement hypothesis is not confirmed by the results relating to cancer deaths, patterns of deaths from other causes suggest it may have some value. For cancer deaths we must await the results of prolonged follow-up of the sample of widowers before drawing final conclusions.

ACKNOWLEDGEMENTS

Thanks are due to Peter Goldblatt, Barbara Scott, Michael Rosato and John Fox for help with and comments on the analyses, and to many OPCS staff for compiling the data on which the paper is based. David Jones was supported by an MRC programme grant at the Social Statistics Research Unit, City University, London, where this work was initiated. The views expressed are not necessarily those of OPCS.

REFERENCES

Berry, G. (1983) The analysis of mortality by the subject-years method. *Biometrics* **39**, 173–184.
Ciocco, A. (1940) On the mortality of husbands and wives. *Hum. Biol.* **12**, 508–513.
Cooper, C. L., Davies Cooper, R. F. and Faragher, E. B. (1986) A prospective study of the

relationship between breast cancer and life events, type A behaviour, social support and coping skills. *Stress Med.* **2**, 271–277.

Craig, T. J. and Brown, G. W. (1984) Life events, meaning and physical illness: a review. In Steptoe, A. and Mathews, A.(ed.) *Health Care and Human Behaviour*, Academic Press, New York.

Evans, E. (1926) *A Psychosocial Study of Cancer*. Dodd-Mead, New York.

Ewertz, M. (1986) Bereavement and breast cancer. *Br. J. Cancer* **53**, 701–703.

Fox, A. J. and Goldblatt, P. O. (1982) *Longitudinal Study: Socio-demographic Mortality Differentials*. Series LS No 1. Office of Population Censuses and Surveys. HMSO, London.

Greer, S. and Morris, T. (1975) Psychological attributes of women who develop breast cancer: A controlled study. *J. Psychosom. Res.* **19**, 147–153.

Holmes, T. H. and Rahe, R. H. (1967) The social readjustment rating scale. *J. Psychosom. Res.* **11**, 213–218.

Horne, R. L. and Picard, R. S. (1980) Psychosocial risk factors for lung cancer. *Psychosom. Med.* **41**, 503–514.

Jacobs, S. and Ostfeld, A. (1979) An epidemiological review of the mortality of bereavement. *Psychosom. Med.* **39**, 344–347.

Jones, D. R. and Goldblatt, P. O. (1987) Heart disease mortality following widowhood: some results from the OPCS Longitudinal Study. *J. Psychosom. Res.* 31, 325–333.

Jones, D. R., Goldblatt, P. O. and Leon, D. A. (1984) Bereavement and cancer: some data on deaths of spouses from the longitudinal study of OPCS. *Br. Med. J.* **289**, 461–464.

Jones, D. R. and Goldblatt, P. O. (1986) Cancer mortality following widow(er)hood: some further results from the OPCS Longitudinal Study. *Stress Med.* **2**, 129–140.

Jones, D. R. and Goldblatt, P. O. (1987) Cause of death in widow(er)s and spouses. *J. Biosoc. Sci.* **19**, 107–121.

Kaplan, B. H., Cassel, J. C. and Gore, S. (1977) Social support and health. *Med. Care* **15**, (Suppl. Part 5), 47–57.

Le Shan, L. (1966) An emotional life-history pattern associated with neoplastic disease. *Ann. NY. Acad. Sci.* **125**, 780–793.

Parkes, C. M. (1986) *Bereavement: Studies of Grief in Adult Life*, 2nd Ed, Tavistock, London.

Parkes, C. M., Benjamin, B. and Fitzgerald, R. G. (1969) Broken heart: A statistical study of increased mortality among widowers. *Br. Med. J.* **1**, 740–743.

Pettingale, K. W. (1985) Towards a psychobiological model of cancer: *Soc. Sci. Med.* **20**, 779–787.

Priestman, T. J., Priestman, S. G. and Bradshaw, C. (1985) Stress and breast cancer. *Br. J. Cancer* **51**, 493–498.

Ramirez, A. (1987) Life events and cancer: conceptual and methodological issues. This volume, pp.53–60. Pergamon, Oxford.

Registrar General (1971) *Registrar General's Statistical Review for England and Wales 1967* Part III. HMSO, London.

Rosch, P. J. (1984) Stress and cancer. In Cooper, C. L. (ed.). *Psychosocial Stress and Cancer*. Wiley, Chichester.

Schleifer, S. J., Keller, S. E., Camerino, M., Thornton, J. C. and Stein, M. (1983) Suppression of lymphocyte stimulation following bereavement.*J. Am. Med. Assoc.* **250**, 374–377.

Snow, H. (1983) *Cancer and the Cancer Process*. Churchill, London.

Susser, M. W. (1981) Widowhood: a situational life stress or a stressful life event? (Editorial). *Am. J. Publ. Health* **71**, 793–795.

Vandenbroucke, J. P. (1982) A shortcut method for calculating the 95% confidence interval of the standardized mortality ratio. *Am. J. Epidemiol.* **115**, 303–304.

World Health Organization (1969) *Manual of International Statistical Classification of Diseases, Injuries and Causes of Death* (8th revision, 1965). WHO, Geneva.

B. Methodology/Theoretical Issues

Measuring Mental Adjustment to Cancer

STEVEN GREER

ABSTRACT

In the burgeoning literature on psychosocial aspects of oncology, scant attention has been paid to the measurement of *mental adjustment to cancer (MAC)* — i.e. the cognitive and behavioural responses of an individual to the diagnosis of cancer. But it is now becoming clear that MAC is important, first because it appears to be related to psychosocial morbidity and, secondly, because evidence from prospective studies suggests (subject to confirmation) that MAC may be a prognostic indicator. Several methods of measuring MAC are described including the recent development of a self-rating scale.

A bad habit which psychiatrists share with sociologists and psychologists is that of inventing obfuscating jargon to describe various aspects of human behaviour. Although the ostensible purpose of this exercise is to develop a scientific language which will aid communication, the effect is often precisely the opposite. In addition to maiming the English language, jargon obscures rather than clarifies meaning and renders psychiatric concepts unintelligible to non-psychiatrists, thereby creating a serious obstacle to inter-disciplinary research. In order to overcome that obstacle, I have tried to avoid "psychobabble" and to describe our research in plain English. This is no mere semantic quibble; our studies of the effect of mental adjustment to cancer on outcome would be pointless unless we were able to communicate the results to surgeons, medical oncologists, radiotherapists and other professionals involved in the care of patients with cancer.

Finding an unambiguous, comprehensive term to encompass the various ways in which patients react psychologically to cancer has proved difficult. Our original term, "psychological responses", was confused by some workers with psychological morbidity. The subsequent heading which we used, namely "mental attitudes" was more specific but still not entirely satisfactory because it excludes behaviour. "Mental adjustment", our current choice, seems a more felicitous term and one which, I hope, will defy attempts at misinterpretation.

In the present context, *mental adjustment* refers to the cognitive and behavioural responses of an individual to the diagnosis of cancer. As defined here, mental adjustment comprises both appraisal (i.e. how the patient perceives the implications of cancer) and the ensuing reactions (i.e. what the patient thinks and does in order to reduce the threat posed by cancer). Affective responses *per se* are not included, but, clearly, certain cognitive and behavioural responses have an affective component. In assigning major importance to cognitive processes, we have been influenced by clinical observations of patients' adjustment to cancer as well as by the cogent theoretical contributions of Lazarus and his colleagues (Lazarus, 1966; Lazarus *et al.*, 1970; Folkman and Lazarus, 1980).

What we have attempted to measure are not the immediate, non-specific stress reactions (Falek & Britton, 1974) seen in newly diagnosed cancer patients (Aitken-Swan, and Easson, 1950; Peck, 1972) but the subsequent, more enduring mental adjustment to cancer. The original study sample comprised a series of women with non-metastatic breast cancer admitted to King's College Hospital. Mental adjustment to cancer was assessed 3 months after operation (in most cases, simple mastectomy) by means of structured interviews. Patients were asked how they regarded the nature and seriousness of their disease and how they had reacted to it. It was found in a preliminary survey that patients' responses could be grouped in four broad, mutually exclusive categories:

(i)   *Stoic acceptance:* a fatalistic outlook, patients accepting the diagnosis.
      Example: "I know I've got cancer, there's nothing I can do, I leave it all to the doctors".

(ii) *Denial:* patients rejected the diagnosis or minimized its seriousness. They did their best to avoid thinking about it, often by keeping busy or concentrating on other problems.
      Example: "The doctors just took my breast off as a precaution".

(iii) *Helplessness/Hopelessness:* patients felt completely engulfed by the knowledge that they had cancer; their lives were disrupted by a constant preoccupation with cancer and impending death.
      Example: "There's nothing they can do, I'm finished".

(v)   *Fighting spirit:* an optimistic attitude accompanied by a search for as much information as possible about cancer with the aim of fighting it.
      Example: "When I was told it was cancer, I thought to myself — I can fight it and defeat it".

These categories of mental adjustment to cancer were subsequently found to be related to outcome at 5 and 10 years follow-up (Greer *et al.*,1979; Pettingale *et al.*, 1985). Patients whose adjustment was categorized as *fighting spirit* or *denial* were significantly more likely to be alive and free from recurrence than patients who responded with *stoic acceptance* or *helplessness-hopelessness*. (Table 1, Figure 1).

TABLE 1. INITIAL PSYCHOLOGICAL RESPONSES TO CANCER BY 5 YEAR OUTCOME

Psychological response 3 months after operation	Outcome at 5 years			
	Alive with no recurrence n = 28	Alive with metastases n = 13	Dead n = 16	Total n = 57
Denial	7	2	1	10
Fighting spirit	8	1	1	10
Stoic acceptance	12	10	10	32
Helplessness/Hopelessness	1	–	4	5

Comparing Recurrence-free survival (n = 28) with Metastatic disease alive or dead (n = 29):
$\chi^2 = 9.0$, d.f.3, P<.03

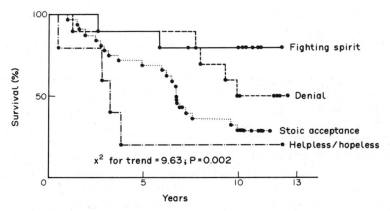

FIG. 1. INITIAL PSYCHOLOGICAL RESPONSES TO CANCER BY 10 YEAR OUTCOME.

What is the most likely explanation for the observed statistical associations between mental adjustment to cancer and subsequent outcome? One possibility is that the various kinds of adjustment merely reflected different stages of cancer and were related to subsequent outcome for that reason. Against this explanation is the fact that patients in each of the four categories of adjustment were found to be similar in terms of all available prognostic factors including clinical stage, histological grade and mammographic appearance. But data regarding two prognostic indicators, viz. lymph node status and oestrogen receptor status were not available when the study began. Consequently, the foregoing explanation cannot be ruled out. There are two other possible explanations for our results:
  (i) mental adjustment to cancer and subsequent outcome are each independently related to a third, unknown factor;
  (ii) mental adjustment to cancer affected 10 year outcome in this series of women with breast cancer.
Whatever the explanation for our results, certain logical implications for further research follow. First, in order to test the hypothesis that mental

adjustment to cancer can influence survival, a new long-term prospective study is required in which all known predictors of outcome are measured. Such an investigation should prove useful. But it could well be, that in 10 years time additional outcome predictors which are unknown today, will be discovered, thereby necessitating yet another cohort study. That process could go on *ad infinitum* (or, rather, until the demise of the interested research group) without providing a definitive answer. This prospect is viewed with less than unrestrained enthusiasm.

A second question arises from our results, namely, can mental adjustment to cancer be altered? The development of a psychological treatment programme designed to alter unfavourable adjustment — particularly *helplessness/hopelessness* — is clearly desirable, first because there is evidence that the degree of psychological distress experienced is related to the kind of mental adjustment to cancer which patients make (Altmaier *et al.*, 1982; Nerenz *et al.*, 1982, Watson *et al.*, 1984) and, secondly, because there is just a possibility that outcome itself could be marginally improved. Evaluation of such a treatment programme will depend crucially on reliable and valid measures of mental adjustment to cancer.

Following our prospective study, Morris and her colleagues embarked on a study which, they hoped, would "illuminate as well as replicate" our results. They studied newly diagnosed patients with early breast cancer, lymphoma and Hodgkin's disease (Morris *et al.*, 1985)

The main aims were to produce operational definitions of cognitive responses to cancer and to devise a reproducible rating method for use in long-term follow-up. They rated responses to questions in a semi-structured interview, gave each response a fuller description with one or more illustrative examples, carried out what they describe as "exhaustive sorting of the responses into broader categories of cognitive response" and, finally, having operationally defined these responses they listed them in a rating manual.

This painstaking investigation describes in detail the manifold responses which patients make. Ten categories of so-called "appraisal statements", 9 categories of "mitigating statements" and 6 categories of "facilitating statements" were identified. In addition to these 25 types of cognitive response, Morris *et al.* listed 29 different behavioural responses. The microscopic detail in which patients' responses were analysed provides valuable descriptive data, but the authors' rather optimistic claim that their method is "practically convenient, flexible and . . . replicable" remains to be tested.

A real replication study of our work was carried out in the U.S. by Di Clemente and Temoshok (1985). Using the same global ratings of mental adjustment to cancer, they conducted semi-structured interviews with a consecutive series of patients with malignant melanoma. Two judges who were blind to patients' medical status, were asked to assign independently each patient to one of the four categories of mental adjustment. Patients were followed up for 18 – 29 months. Their study provides some confirmatory evidence for our results: *stoic acceptance* in female patients and *helplessness/hopelessness* in males were found to be significant predictors of disease progression based on Clark's level of invasion and tumour thickness.

Di Clemente and Temoshok then proceeded to derive a quantitative measure for each of the four adjustment categories by asking judges to (i) identify actual words and phrases which were valuable in assigning patients to a particular category and (ii) rate how intensely each word or phrase represented the adjustment category. Words which showed "high reliability between the judges' intensity ratings were used to anchor a four-point numerical scale". The development of this quantitative measure from the original global ratings appears to be a useful advance in methodology. Its application in other studies of cancer patients is awaited with interest.

One prospective study (Cassileth *et al.*, 1985), also from the U.S., has failed to confirm the statistical correlation between hopelessness and outcome. In that study, patients with mainly advanced cancers of the breast, lung, stomach, bowel and pancreas were followed up to determine the length of survival. Hopelessness was measured by the Beck scale (Beck *et al.*, 1974). This investigation is not comparable with our study because (i) a different measure of *helplessness/hopelessness* was used, (ii) the other categories of mental adjustment were not assessed, and (iii) the patients were suffering from more advanced cancers.

Although the global clinical ratings of broad categories of mental adjustment to cancer have provided some stimulating results, this method has two distinct disadvantages. The criteria for assessment are descriptive and imprecise, making replication studies difficult. Moreover, the method requires skilful, sensitive, trained interviewers and takes at least 1 hour for each patient; it is therefore impractical to use in investigations of large numbers of patients attending busy oncology units. Clearly, a quantitative measure is required. With this aim in view, we are developing a self-rating questionnaire — the MAC (mental adjustment to cancer) *scale* (Watson *et al.*, 1988). This scale consists of items which are based on patients' verbatim responses obtained in our previous studies. So far, 235 patients with various types and stages of cancer attending King's College Hospital and the Royal Marsden Hospital have completed the MAC scale, which is also being completed by patients with cancers at two centres in the United States.

It may be safely concluded that, during the next few years increasing attention will be focused on the study of mental adjustment to cancer.

One reason for this is that with greater numbers of patients surviving cancer (not to mention cancer treatments), there is growing interest in the survivors' quality of life of which mental adjustment to cancer is an integral part. The other principle reason is that recent research suggests the possibility that mental adjustment to cancer may have prognostic significance. Research in this new area is not merely a matter of academic interest; its over-riding aim is therapeutic. We are compellingly reminded of that aim when we read the eloquent accounts written by some of our patients. Among such accounts, none is more poignant than the recent, painfully honest testimony of a woman who developed maxillo-facial cancer. Christine Piff (1985) describes the reaction to the diagnosis as follows:

"The room was dark, there was nobody there. 'You're not going to let cancer beat you, are you?' A voice in my head answered: 'No, I won't give up for some lousy old cells that I don't want. I'll fight with every ounce of strength I have".

It is the need to provide effective help for Christine Piff and others like her, that provides the most important reason for the rigorous scientific study of mental adjustment to cancer.

ACKNOWLEDGEMENTS

I am grateful to Mrs. Faith Scott-Elliot whose generosity enabled our research to proceed, to my gifted colleagues Keith Pettingale and Maggie Watson for their invaluable collaboration, to Maria Wong, our secretary, for her unfailing patience and good humoured efficiency, and, finally, to the patients who were kind enough to allow me to interview them at a particularly stressful time in their lives.

My thanks are also due to the editor of the *Lancet* and its publishers for permission to reproduce tables and parts of the text previously published in that journal.

REFERENCES

Aitken-Swan, J. and Easson, E. C. (1959) Reactions of cancer patients on being told their diagnosis. *Br. Med. J.* **1**, 779–783.

Altmaier, E. M., Ross, W. E. and Moore, K. (1982) A pilot investigation of the psychologic functioning of patients with anticipatory vomiting. *Cancer* **49**, 201–204.

Beck, A. T., Weissman, A., Lester, D. and Trexler, L. (1974) The measurement of pessimism: the hopelessness scale. *J. Consult. Clin. Psychol.* **42**, 861–865.

Cassileth, B. R., Lusk, E.J., Miller, D. S., Brown, L.L and Miller, C. (1985) Psychosocial correlates of survival in advanced malignant disease? *N. Engl. J. Med.* **312**, 1551–1555.

Di Clemente, R. J. and Temoshok, L. (1985) Psychological adjustment to having cutaneous malignant melanoma as a predictor of follow-up clinical status. *Psychosom. Med,* **47**, 81.

Falek, A. and Britton, S. (1974) Phases in coping: the hypothesis and its implications. *Soc. Biol.* **21** (1), 219–239.

Folkman, S. and Lazarus, R. S. (1980) An analysis of coping in a middle-aged community sample. *J. Health Soc. Behav.* **21**, 1–7.

Greer, S., Morris, T. and Pettingale, K. W. (1979) Psychological response to breast cancer: effect on outcome. *Lancet* **ii**, 785–787.

Lazarus, R. S. (1966) *Psychological Stress and the Coping Process.* McGraw-Hill, New York.

Lazarus, R. S., Averill, J. R. and Opton, E. M. (1970) Towards a cognitive theory of emotion. In *Feelings and Emotions* pp.207–232, Academic Press, New York. (Arnold, M. B. ed.)

Morris, T., Blake, S. and Buckley, M. (1985) Development of a method for rating cognitive responses to a diagnosis of cancer. *Soc. Sci. Med.* **20**, 795–802.

Nerenz, D. R., Leventhal, H and Love, R. R. (1982) Factors contributing to emotional distress during cancer chemotherapy. *Cancer* **50**, 1020–1027.

Peck A. (1972) Emotional reactions to having cancer *Am. J. Roentgen. Radium Ther. Nuc. Med.* **114**, 591–599.

Pettingale, K. W., Morris, T., Greer, S. and Haybittle, J. L. (1985) Mental attitudes to cancer: an additional prognostic factor. *Lancet* **i**, 750.

Piff, C. (1985) *Lets Face It.* Gollancz, London.

Watson, M., Greer, S., Blake, S. and Shrapnell, K. (1984) Reaction to a diagnosis of breast cancer – relationship between denial, delay and rates of psychological morbidity. *Cancer* **53**, 2008–2012..

Watson, M., Greer, S., Young, J., Inayat, Q., Burgess, C., Robertson, B. (1988) Development of a questionnaire measure of adjustment to cancer: The MAC Scale. *Psychological Medicine*, **18**, in press.

Life Events and Cancer: Conceptual and Methodological Issues

AMANDA J. RAMIREZ

ABSTRACT

There is anecdotal evidence dating from the 18th century supporting a causal link between stressful life experiences and cancer, more recent systematic research has been less conclusive.

The contradictory nature of the evidence may be understood in terms of a number of conceptual and methodological issues relevant to this area of research. These include the meaning of the life experience, the type of data collection (respondent or investigator based instruments), the nature of the control population and the dating of tumour onset and progression.

A psychobiological model of cancer incorporating adverse life events is proposed. A study designed to test this model is described.

There is a growing body of substantive research which supports the relationship between life events and the development of certain physical illnesses, including myocardial infarction, (Connolly, 1976) subarachnoid haemorrhage, (Penrose, 1972), painful gastrointestinal disorders, (Craig and Brown, 1984) appendicitis, (Creed, 1981) multiple sclerosis (Grant, 1985) and diabetes mellitus (Robinson and Fuller, 1985). To date, evidence for the link between life events and the onset and progression of cancer is less conclusive.

The 18th and 19th century medical literature contains various references to these associations, including repeated observations made by eminent physicians among them Richard Guy, James Paget and Herbert Snow. Gendron in 1701 reported two cases.

Case One

"Mrs Emerson upon the death of her daughter underwent great affliction and perceived her breast to swell, it broke out in a most inveterate cancer . . . she had always enjoyed a perfect state of health".

Case Two

"The wife of the Mate of a ship (who was taken sometime ago by the French and put in prison) was thereby so much affected that her breast began to swell and soon after broke out in a desperate cancer . . . she had never before had any complaint in her breast".

LIFE EVENTS AND THE ONSET OF CANCER

In a review in 1959 of 75 studies on psychological factors in the development of malignancy LeShan concluded that "the most consistently recorded relevant psychological factor had been the loss of a major emotional relationship prior to the first noted symptoms of the neoplasms".

More recent systematic research of the relationship between life events and the onset of cancer has yielded less consistent findings.

Two epidemiological studies have failed to demonstrate a correlation between one major type of loss event, death of a spouse, and the subsequent onset of cancer. Jones *et al.* (1984) using data from the longitudinal study of the Office of Population Censuses and Surveys in the United Kingdom found only slight evidence of greater than expected registration of cancer following conjugal bereavement. Possible reasons for this are firstly the small numbers of people in the population with the combination of events that were of interest and secondly the overall unreliability of cancer registration in the United Kingdom. Similar results were obtained by Ewertz (1986) using the Danish Cancer Registry which has data on virtually all cancer cases in Denmark.

Six clinical studies of women with breast cancer have failed to reveal a significant association between the onset of cancer and antecedent stressful events (Muslin *et al.*, 1966; Snell and Graham, 1971; Schonfield, 1975; Greer and Morris, 1975; Priestman *et al.*, 1985; Cooper and Davies-Cooper, 1986). Similar negative findings emerge from a study of monozygotic twins discordant for haematological malignancies (Smith *et al.*, 1984) and from an investigation of patients with lung cancer (Grissom *et al.*, 1975).

In contrast four studies, which looked at patients with lung cancer (Horne and Picard, 1979), gastric carcinoma (Lehrer, 1980) breast cancer (Cheang and Cooper, 1985) and children with a number of different cancers (Jacobs and Charles, 1980) respectively, all found a significant correlation between the onset of the cancer and preceding life events.

The clinical investigations cited all fulfill the basic requirement of being controlled studies of unselected series of patients with documented neoplastic disease. Despite this they are flawed with conceptual and methodological shortcomings which might explain the contradictory nature of their results.

The meaning of life events

Perhaps one of the most important conceptual weaknesses common to the majority of these studies is their measurement of life events according to the propensity of those events to produce *change and disruption* rather than their *undesirability*. Eight of the twelve studies used instruments designed to measure adjustment or change such as the Holmes and Rahe (1967) Schedule of Recent Experiences or variants of it.

Scrutiny of the early literature suggests, however that it is the undesirable and threatening nature of events which is important. In particular it is those events that involve loss that are most pertinent. In order to test the hypothesis that severely threatening events which involve loss, are causally related to the development of cancer, an alternative approach to life event measurement, which attempts to deal with the meaning for the individual, is required. Such an approach is embraced in the Bedford College Life Events and Difficulties Schedule designed by Brown and Harris (1978). In this the measurement of life events is described as contextual in recognition of the fact that specific meaning is dealt with by taking into account the person's biography and the circumstances surrounding a particular event.

It is noteworthy that the Horne and Picard study of lung cancer (1979) which did inquire about recent losses (including death of a spouse, divorce, separation, death of a parent or a sibling) and probed about them for their contextual significance in a semi-structured interview did demonstrate a positive correlation between life events and the subsequent onset of cancer.

Method of data collection

A methodological weakness found in nine of the 12 studies is the use of respondent-based methods to collect data, mainly standardized questionnaires which included vague items that left it to the subject to decide on the criteria for inclusion of an event. This introduces a serious potential for bias and unreliability.

For example the tendency to over-report by those subjects who knew they had cancer and whose decision to include events would be influenced by their attempt to make sense of their illness. The so-called "effort after meaning" phenomenon.

Conversely, in those studies in which subjects did not yet know their diagnosis, although the bias due to self-reporting would be brought under some degree of control, the general inaccuracy and insensitivity of the respondent-based approach would lead to a low association.

More controversially but perhaps more relevantly is the possibility that the behaviour pattern described by a number of different workers (including Greer and Watson, 1985; Temoshok, 1985) as being typical of cancer patients, and which involves suppression of emotional responses particularly anger might lead to the consistent under-reporting of adverse events using this method of data collection.

Amanda J. Ramirez

The Life Events and Difficulties Schedule attempts to rule out the bias due to self-reporting by using a semi-structured interview to gather as coherent and as full account as possible of any incident which might be relevant to the research enquiry. A set of previously developed rules and detailed questioning is used to decide whether or not an event is to be included. By ignoring self reports about meaning, various potential sources of bias stemming from the respondent can be ruled out and by using raters who are ignorant of such self reports potential bias stemming from the investigator is brought under control. This approach also avoids any judgement about likely causal links between the events and disorder by ensuring that the raters who make the contextual rating do not know whether the event was followed by the onset of an illness.

Control groups

The nature of the control populations used in the clinical studies provides a further source of methodological error. They were mainly derived from in-patient populations, most of the control patients had organic pathology. In the case of the breast cancer studies the controls were mainly women with benign breast lumps (themselves risk factors in breast cancer). Snell and Graham's study of breast cancer patients actually included women with other malignant disease in the control groups. It seems likely, in view of the documented effect of stressful life events on consulting behaviour, physical symptoms and certain physical diseases, that patients in these control populations would have increased incidence of life events prior to their admission compared to the general population and therefore their use as a control group might mask any correlation between life events and the onset of cancer in the study group.

Dating the onset of cancer

The outstanding weakness in these studies looking at the role of life events in the aetiology of cancer is their inability to date accurately the onset of cancer in order to ensure that the life events preceded that onset. In reality the correlation observed in these studies is between life events and the *clinical* onset of the malignancy and it is possible that many of the stressful life events were occurring in the context of early undetected malignant disease. Indeed, it is also possible that those life events that did genuinely antedate the onset of tumour growth were not ascertained because they occurred outside the time period under scrutiny.

LIFE EVENTS AND THE PROGRESSION OF CANCER

The role of life events in the prognosis of an already established cancer has received much less attention. Jones in his epidemiological study of cancer registration and death rates following widow(er)hood found only a weak suggestion of increased mortality in those who suffered a conjugal bereavement after registration of their cancer compared with those who did not. His more detailed analysis of post widow(er)hood mortality (Jones and Goldblatt, 1986) demonstrates that such excesses as do occur are to be seen in 6 months or more after bereavement. This could be taken as weak evidence in support of the association between bereavement and excess mortality from cancer, with a relatively long interval between widow(er)hood and death from cancer of the widow(er). Further follow-up of this cohort might yield more information about mortality from a disease with a potentially long latent interval.

Until now, therefore, the evidence relating to the role of life events in the aetiology and promotion of cancer has been contradictory. Inability to date the onset of tumour growth means that the role of adverse life events in the aetiology of cancer cannot yet be studied. The progress of an already diagnosed tumour is, however, more amenable to measurement. The close clinical and investigatory scrutiny of cancer patients facilitates preclinical diagnosis of recurrence and the disease spread.

ONE APPROACH: THE RATIONALE AND DESIGN OF A CASE CONTROLLED STUDY

It is with due attention to all these conceptual and methodological issues that a study looking at the influence of adverse life events and difficulties on the prognosis of breast cancer is currently in progress at Guy's Hospital, London. The hypotheses that this investigation addresses are based on a psychobiological approach to cancer promotion. Namely, that the progress of an established cancer depends on the intrinsic properties of the tumour and on the efficacy of the homeostatic controls which regulate cell growth and function. It is not posited that psychosocial factors are either necessary or sufficient promoting agents, but that through their interaction with biological homeostatic mechanisms they contribute to the progress of the cancer and thus to the development of the recurrences.

The study is designed to test three specific hypotheses, first that adverse life events are causally related to the development of recurrences and it is the severely threatening life events and major difficulties which involve loss or threat of loss that are most important. Secondly, that other psychosocial factors, namely patients cognitive coping strategies and social support, have a mediating influence on the relationship between adverse life experiences and biological disease outcome. Thirdly, that psychological morbidity, in particular depression, acts as a marker or manifestation of the underlying biological process which leads to disease progression. This last notion is derived from Murphy and Brown's (1980) model of the relationship between life events and the onset of illness, which proposes that stressful events are only important in so far as they lead to an affective disorder which in itself is the main risk factor for subsequent organic disease.

The study is a retrospective comparison of a group of women with early breast cancer who have developed their first recurrence, with a control group of women who also have early breast cancer but who remain in remission (according to clinical and investigatory criteria). The two groups are compared with respect to the presence of life events, social support and coping strategies and matched on a pairwise basis according to socio-demographic, clinical, physical and pathological criteria. The women are interviewed on one occasion: for those who have developed a recurrence they are seen as soon as possible after its detection.

At interview, socio-demographic details are obtained. Adverse life experiences are assessed using the Bedford College instrument. The information is collected for the time period from diagnosis of the cancer to recurrence and the equivalent disease-free interval in the control group.

Cognitive coping strategies are assessed using a semi-structured interview designed by Morris *et al.* (1985) to elicit patients understanding and evaluation of their cancer diagnosis and the cognitive and behavioural strategies they employ in order to cope with the implications.

Social support is assessed looking particularly at the active emotional and practical support provided in the context of a confiding relationship. The assessment is derived from the Self Evaluation and Social Support Schedule (O'Connor and Brown, 1984).

Psychiatric morbidity is assessed using the Present State Examination constructed by Wing *et al.* in 1974.

The design of this study answers many of the criticisms discussed earlier.

Accurate dating and assessment of life experiences is achieved using the Bedford College Instrument.

Early and accurate dating of recurrences is made possible by the very regular surgical follow-up of the women attending the Breast Unit — 6–12 weekly for the first 5 years after diagnosis. The follow-up involves regular physical examination, blood tests and radioisotope scans. Recurrences are diagnosed on the basis of these clinical and investigatory assessments and where possible confirmed pathologically. The date of recurrence is taken as the date of the first symptoms pertaining to that recurrence or, if no symptoms are complained of, the date on which the clinical abnormalities are detected.

Awareness that the influence of psychosocial variables in the development of cancer may not be great, means that in order to discern this contribution meticulous control for clinical and pathological variables is essential. To this end each woman who developed a recurrence is matched with regard to the size of her tumour, the tumour pathology, number of axillary lymph nodes involved and menopausal status and disease-free interval.

Finally, this approach allows a detailed scrutiny of the type of loss events and difficulties which may be important in the development of recurrence in breast cancer. There is for example an indication that the most important events and difficulties are those which reinforce for a woman with breast cancer the implications of her disease, either in terms of its threat to her mortality or loss of femininity. An example of the first type of event would be the death from cancer of a *confidante* and an example of the second type would be infidelity of a husband in the context of poor sexual adjustment following mastectomy. There is also a suggestion that such implication-reinforcing events have most impact on women who cope with their breast cancer using strategies of denial. In the face of such events, the coping strategies break down, the implication of having cancer can no longer be denied and so the women are left overwhelmed by its full adverse psychological impact. These ideas remain speculative, but nevertheless testable within the design of the study.

The role of adverse life experiences in the prognosis of cancer remains uncertain. The design of this retrospective case-controlled study should provide a valid, reliable, time-limited and economical first step in improving our understanding this relationship. Evidence from this work may be used as the basis for subsequent large scale prospective studies. Improvement in tumour technology facilitating the accurate dating of onset of malignant growth will allow the role of life events in the aetiology of cancers to be subjected to similar scrutiny.

REFERENCES

Brown, G. H. and Harris, T. (1978) Social origins of depression. *A Study of Psychosocial Disorder in Women* Tavistock Publications, London.

Cheang, A. and Cooper, C. L. (1985) Psychosocial factors in breast cancer. *Stress Med.* **1**, 11–24.

Connolly, J. (1976) Life events before myocardial infarction. *J. Hum. Stress* **2**, (4), 3–7.

Cooper, C. L. and Davies-Cooper, R. F. (1986) A prospective study of the relationship between breast cancer and life events, type of behavior, social support and coping skills. *Stress Med.* **2**, 271–277.

Craig T. K. J. and Brown, G. W. (1984) Goal frustration and life events in the aetiology of painful gastrointestinal disorders. *J. Psychosom. Research* **28**, 411–421.

Creed, F. H. (1981) Life events and appendectomy. *Lancet* i, 1381–1385.

Ewertz, M. (1986) Bereavement and breast cancer. *Br. J. Cancer* **53**, 701–703.

Gendon, D. (1701) *Enquiries into the Nature, Knowledge and Cure of Cancers.* London.

Grant, I. (1985) The social environment and neurological disease. *Adv. Psychosom. Med.* **13**, 26–48.

Greer, S. and Morris, T. (1975) Psychological attributes of women who develop breast cancer: a controlled study. *J. Psychosom. Res.* **19**, 147-53.

Greer, S. and Watson, M. (1985) Toward a psychobiological model of cancer: psychological considerations. *Soc. Sci. Med.* **20**(8), 773–777.

Grissom, J., Weiner, B. and Weiner, E. (1975) Psychological correlations of cancer. *J. Counsell. Clin. Psycholo.* **43**,113.

Holmes, T. H. and Rahe, R. H. (1967) The social readjustment scale. *J. Psychosom. Res.* **11**, 213–218.

Horne, R. L. and Picard, R. S. (1979) Psychosocial risk factors for lung cancer. *Psychosom. Med.* **41**, 503, 514.

Jacobs, T. J. and Charles, E. (1980) Life events and occurrence of cancer in children. *Pyschosom. Med.* **42**(1), 11–24.

Jones, D. R. and Goldblatt, P. O. (1986) Cancer mortality following widow(er)hood: Some further results from the OPCS longitudunal study. *Stress Med.* **2**, 129–140.

Jones, D. R., Goldblatt, P. O. and Leon, D. A. (1984) Bereavement and cancer, some data on deaths of spouses from the longitudinal study of the Office of Population Censuses and Surveys. *Br. Med. J.* **289**, 461–464.

Lehrer, S. (1980) Life change and gastric cancer. *Psychosom. Med.* **42**(5), 499–502.

LeShan, L. (1959) Psychological states as factors in the development of malignant diseases; A critical review. *J. Natl Cancer Inst.* **22**, 1–18.

Morris, T., Blake, S. and Buckley, M. (1985) Development of a method for rating cognitive responses to a diagnosis of cancer. *Soc. Sci. Med.* **20**(8), 795.

Murphy, E. and Brown, G. W. (1980) Life events, psychiatric disturbance and physical illness. *Br. J. Psychiat.* **136**, 326–338.

Muslin, H. L., Gyarfas, K. and Pieper, W. (1966) Separation experience and cancer of the breast.

Ann. N.Y. Acad. Sci. **125**, 802–806.

O'Connor, P and Brown, G. W. (1984) Supportive relationships: fact or fancy? *J. Soc. Pers. Relat.* **1**, 159–195.

Penrose, R. J. J. (1972) Life events before subarachnoid haemorrhage. *J. Psychosom. Res.* **16**, 329–333.

Priestman, T. J., Priestman, S. G. and Bradshaw, C. (1985) Stress and breast cancer. *Br. J. Cancer* **5**, 493–498

Robinson, N. and Fuller, J. H. (1985) Role of life events and difficulties in the onset of diabetes mellitus. *J. Psychosom. Res.* **29**(6), 583–91.

Schonfield, J. (1975) Psychological and life experience differences between Israeli women with benign and cancerous breast lesions. *J. Psychosom. Res.* **43**, 117–125.

Smith, C. K., Harrison, S. D., Ashworth, C., Montiano, D., Davis, A. and Fefer, A. (1984) Life change and onset of cancer in identical twins. *J. Psychosom. Res.* **28**, 525–532.

Snell, L. and Graham, S. (1971) Social trauma as related to cancer of the breast. *Br. J. Cancer* **25**, 721–734.

Temoshok, L. (1985) Biopsychological studies and cutaneous malignant melanoma. *Soc. Sci. Med.* **20**(8), 833-840.

Wing, J. K., Cooper, J. E. and Sartorious, N. (1974) *Measurement and Classification of Psychiatric Symptoms.* Cambridge University Press, Cambridge.

Quality of Life: Conceptual and Theoretical Considerations

J. C. J. M. DE HAES

ABSTRACT

In this paper attention will be given, in the first place, to the function of the concept quality of life, especially in oncology, in the second place, to the meaning of the concept and the choices made when defining the concept and, in the third place, to the factors contributing to the quality of life as suggested by different authors.

Function and use of the concept quality of life

The concept quality of life became increasingly popular in recent years. For example, in a recent editorial of the British Medical Journal, the importance of including quality of life as an end-point in clinical cancer trials was stressed (Brinkley, 1985). Within the Index Medicus the concept was not used as a subject until 1975. In that year it said: "quality of life, see under philosophy". In 1977 it became a separate subject. In Fig. 1 the number of titles in the Index Medicus in which quality of life or quality of survival is mentioned is shown. As will be evident, there is an increase in the number of publications and, thus, we may assume in the scientific use of quality of life.

It seems as though the use of the concept quality of life is becoming commercially attractive. In one of this year's issues of the journal Cancer, two advertisements on drugs enhancing the quality of life in palliative treatment could be found.

Apparently, the concept 'quality of life' is useful. However, the question is what function it has in the debate on oncology care and in oncology research. It is used by care-givers to clarify that the patients' well-being is an objective of cancer care: the quantity along with the quality of survival. Thus generally speaking the function is, to differentiate between the effect of cancer and cancer treatment on the length of survival on the one hand, and on the functioning of the patient, on the other hand.

In oncological research it is used to study the impact of cancer and treatment on personal functioning. This may be done descriptively, to enhance patient information and counselling. Most often, quality of life studies are used to compare the impact of different treatment modalities

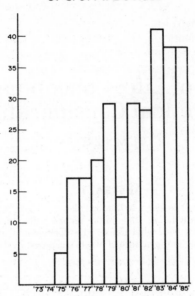

FIG. 1. NUMBER OF TITLES IN WHICH
QUALITY OF LIFE (SURVIVAL) IS
MENTIONED IN THE INDEX-MEDICUS

on the functioning of patients. Thus treatment policy can be influenced by quality of life research (Bush, 1979). For instance two treatment regimes may be expected to be equally effective with respect to survival or other medical parameters, but to have an unequal impact on the quality of life. Some examples of this kind of research are: studies on the effectiveness of analogous cytostatics, of a lower number of chemotherapy courses, or of the effectiveness of less mutilating surgical modalities such as breast-conserving treatment. A further question posed, is whether the impact of a specific treatment on survival outweighs the disadvantages of the same treatement.

People wonder whether the burden placed on the patient by the treatment is worth the short gain in survival. In this case, studies are used in weighing up the costs and benefits of treatment. This research question is of utmost importance in palliative treatment.

In any case, the function of quality of life research is primarily to study or indicate the impact of cancer treatment on the different aspects of personal functioning of patients and eventually to be able to include considerations with respect to the quality of life in medical decision making.

Defining the concept quality of life

So far, the function of quality of life seems relevant. However, what does quality of life mean? The answer to this question is of importance as the results of studies on the quality of life will, to a great extent, depend on the conceptualization of the concept.

There is no agreement on the content of the concept or the way to conceptualize quality of life. Surprisingly, when reviewing the literature, the choice of variables, intended to measure quality of life turned out to be seldom or never made explicit (de Haes and van Knippenberg, 1985). Moreover, different authors used rather different operationalizations, although they attempted to measure the same concept. Most authors did include some measurement of physical functioning, such as the occurrence of physical symptoms and side effects of treatment. Most authors included also the activity level of patients and instruments that measure in some way or other, psychological distress.

The global evaluation of life was often included. However, social and material consequences of illness are only measured occasionally. Structural functioning, the way a person is involved in and participates in society, is not measured in any of these instruments (Hörnquist, 1982).

As the choice of variables is often not justified, it may be assumed that this choice is made arbitrarily. However, to reach meaningful and controllable results in quality of life studies, the conceptualization has to be elaborated. Thus, the question is, what is the meaning of the concept quality of life and how is it to be defined.

We have reviewed a number of definitions of quality of life in an earlier paper (de Haes and van Knippenberg, 1985). Two issues were evolving from the comparison of these definitions. The first issue is, whether quality of life is considered an objective judgement or a subjective evaluation. This means, in practical terms, who is to judge the situation of the patient? Up to 1979 this was done mostly by physicians, using the Karnofsky or Zubrod Index (Bardelli and Saracci, 1978). Nowadays this Index is still considered a measure of quality of life in some studies (Bakker *et al.*, 1984). Also, in medical decision making, using decision trees, physicians may judge the extent to which life is worth less to the patient, in order to determine the so called quality adjusted survival (Weinstein and Fineberg, 1980). Some years ago an index was constructed by Spitzer and others (1981), on which the physicians judge the global evaluation of the quality of life of patients. In their study, they compared, for validation reasons, the judgement of patients and physicians on this same index. Although the correlation was rather high, the patients' judgement turned out to be consistently more positive than the physician's. Presumably they do not agree on quality of life. Perhaps something different is being judged.

This finding can be explained. In the first place physicians will tend to judge the situation more or less from a medical point of view. They will observe those side effects of treatment visible in the medical setting, but not the impact of treatment on, for example, family life or the material

```
┌─────────────────────────────────────┐
│                                      │
│        Quality of life is            │
│                                      │
│     the subjective evaluation        │
│                                      │
│        of life as a whole            │
│                                      │
└─────────────────────────────────────┘
```

FIG. 2.
DEFINITION OF
QUALITY OF LIFE

condition of the patient. In the second place, the way in which a situation is experienced is strictly personal. No other person can know exactly how a patient experiences his or her situation. Nobody but the patient can be considered able to weigh satisfactions and dissatisfactions (de Groot, 1978). Therefore, decisions made on the basis of these judgements may only be reached by the patient as others cannot judge the costs and benefits. Based on this reasoning, quality of life is considered to be a subjective evaluation. Fortunately, most instruments developed to measure quality of life in recent years take this point of view (de Haes *et al.*, 1983; Padilla *et al.*, 1983; Priestman and Baum, 1976; Schipper *et al.*, 1984; Selby *et al.*, 1984).

A second issue is, whether the evaluation is related only to certain aspects of life, or to life as a whole. If some areas are considered to be important to the quality of life, the question is, which areas are to be considered relevant. If a patient is asked which aspects of life he or she thinks relevant, he may ask: "relevant to what?". The answer will be, logically: "to life as a whole". Therefore, it seems logical to consider life as a whole.

From a common sense point of view, the process of evaluating the quality of life, may be compared to the judgement made about, for example, a bottle of wine. A person may buy a bottle because of the price or because of the colour he wants for a specific dinner. If afterwards he liked the taste, and the atmosphere of the evening was good, he will be satisfied with the bottle and say the wine was nice. He will have integrated certain aspects into a global evaluation. Likewise, as Szalaï (1980) suggests, if you ask a person "How are you?" and this person wants to give an honest answer, he will integrate certain aspects of life and be able to say it is good or bad at a specific moment.

Therefore, quality of life must be seen as an evaluation of life as a whole. It is not the same as the quality of an aspect of life like the quality of physical functioning or the support system.

To summarize, it seems preferable, to define quality of life as a subjective evaluation concerning life as a whole (see Fig. 2). If this definition is taken as a starting point, it has implications for quality of life research with cancer patients. First, starting from this definition, it is possible to see how the consequences of treatment and disease will be integrated in the evaluation of life as a whole. For example the emphasis given to different side effects may be different. It is not only important to know that patients are suffering from side effects, but also to what extent they interfere with their lives. The amount of emphasis given to different consequences of treatment can be investigated by relating these, statistically, to the global evaluation of life.

Second, by choosing this definition, it is possible to draw comparisons. In the research literature relating to quality of life of the general population, quality of life is seen as a global concept (Campbell *et al.*, 1976; Andrews and Withey, 1976; Michalos, 1980). Therefore, using this approach cancer studies can be related to studies on the population at large. Comparisons can be drawn and, thus, what is specific and what is comparable in the condition of having cancer and being treated for other diseases can be investigated. Thus, we gain more insight into the consequences of illness and cancer treatment.

Factors leading to quality of life

After having chosen a definition, the point to be raised concerns which factors play a role in the evaluation of life as a whole, or, more down to earth, what leads to a better or a poorer quality of life. Is it the condition of having cancer, the treatment given or, are other things involved?

To start with, the assumption that cancer and cancer treatments are having an impact on the quality of life underlies all quality of life research in cancer.

In our review of the literature, we found that differences between cancer patients and others are less clear than is generally assumed (de Haes & van Knippenberg, 1985). However, many of these studies referred to long term survivors and the hypothesis can not yet be rejected. In a study on the quality of life of early breast cancer patients we found that the global evaluation of life was more positive 1½ years after surgery then it was at 1 year after surgery (de Haes *et al.*, 1986). Therefore, we concluded that the experience of illness had a negative impact on the overall evaluation of life.

From the literature on the population at large it becomes evident, that quality of life is an aggregation of the evaluation of different aspects of life (Andrews and Witney, 1976; Michalos, 1980). A model, suggested by Hörnquist (1982) clarifies the aspects considered relevant in the experiences of disease, and this model does seem to be exhaustive. It suggests aspects of human functioning (physical, psychological, social, activities, material and structural) which may be affected by the illness independently. Cancer and cancer treatments have, obviously, an impact on these aspects of life. Physical functioning is impaired after

treatment and in progressive disease. Psychological consequences have
been described extensively by different authors (Pruyn, 1983). Social
consequences have been reviewed by Wortman (1984). The patient's
activity level is often lowered: daily activities as well as specific role
activities are difficult to perform in some stages of illness. Financial
consequences are often underestimated. Patients need extra money for
travelling, diet and household expenses. Also, their income may be
lower. Structural functioning refers to the participation in society.
Cancer patients have been described, in one Dutch study, as having less
interest and being less well integrated into society (van Doorn *et al.*,
1983). It should be noted, however, that some positive feelings may result
from the patient's confrontation with the disease. Some patients report
being more conscious about living and enjoying their days than they used
to be (van Doorn *et al.*, 1983; Yalom, 1980). For others the shared
experience and confrontation with the possible end of life may lead to
more intense or intimate relations with their partner and others
(Meyerowitz *et al.*, 1983).

Thus, cancer and cancer treatments influence the functioning and the
evaluation of different aspects of life. These may be integrated
differently into a global judgement of life as a whole.

Finally, the most complicated part is, that the way people experience
life and their personal functioning, is influenced by factors independent
from the objective illness situation. This is as true for cancer as it is for
suffering from influenza. In the latter situation patients do, obviously,
react in a different manner. Some people may enjoy staying in bed for a
couple of days and being cared for. Others feel guilty and have difficulty
with not being able to work for example. The same is true for cancer
patients. In the study by Coates *et al.* (1983) patients who had higher
extraversion scores reported that the physical and non-physical side
effects of chemotherapy were less important to them. Likewise, in the
study of Mettlin *et al.* (1983), dimensions of the quality of life turned out to
be related to the age and the sex of the patient. In studies on the quality of
life of cancer patients, personal factors have frequently not been
studied. These do, however, exert an influence on the experience of the
disease. Therefore, as shown in Fig. 3 the final quality of life model
should include factors other than disease related ones if we want to have
insight into the process of evaluating life with illness.

There has not been much research performed on personal factors
contributing to the quality of life of cancer patients. However, based on
the literature and the theories forwarded in other fields some possible
ways in which personal mechanisms and characteristics could play a
role in the evaluation of life quality are presented.

First, quality of life is evaluated by the person concerned. This
evaluation is, therefore, the outcome of a cognitive process. This

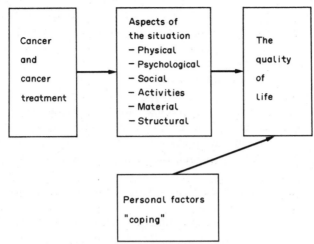

FIG. 3. A QUALITY OF LIFE MODEL

cognitive process may be influenced by mechanisms used to restructure the experience of the situation in order to make life more bearable. This may be seen as a type of cognitive coping. Three ways in which this cognitive restructuring may take place have been suggested in the quality of life literature. With respect to the quality of life of cancer patients, Calman (1984) has suggested that the evaluation of life is, partly, the result of the aspiration level of the individual. This hypothesis is in accordance with suggestions by other authors (Campbell, 1976; Michalos, 1985). Cancer patients may develop different aspirations as they get involved in the disease process.

Patients may reduce their expectations. For example, someone may lower his ambitions in relation to work and in this way stay more satisfied with life. Thus, the gap between aspirations and the situation is narrowed and the quality of life may stay the same.

Another way of restoring quality of life through cognitive processes is by social comparison. Patients may look at someone whose condition is worse than their own and think that it could have been worse, so it is judged to be relatively better. In this way they may think their life is not that bad. In a recent Dutch study by van den Borne and Pruyn (1985) it was found that many cancer patients use their contact with other patients to reduce their negative feelings about their illness. In studies on the quality of life of the population at large, social comparison turned out to be strongly related to the evaluation of life as a whole (Michalos, 1985).

From the adaptation level theory suggested by Helson and Bevan (1967), it may be deduced that negative experiences give people a different reference point. Thus, when people felt bad one day, they would be more positive if they felt a little less bad the next day. This feeling may lead to a more positive evaluation than it would have, had they not had these negative experiences beforehand. Patients' judgements of the situation are relative to what had occurred to them in the past.

Thus, cognitive methods of restructuring the objective situation into a subjective opinion about this situation seem to be involved in perceptions of quality of life. They explain the way in which people evaluate their lives. Also, some factors in their personal life seem to make some patients better able to restore their quality of life than others. This may also be seen as a form of coping with the adversities of cancer. Patients may have, as Calman (1984) suggests, the energy to improve their situation more adequately.

The question remains of which factors make some patients more able to handle their situation than others.

As suggested earlier, there is little research in those personal factors which enhance the quality of life of cancer patients. Studies by Mettlin *et al.* (1983) and Coates *et al.* (1983), indicated that the patient's age and sex on the one hand, and neuroticism and extraversion on the other hand, are related to the way in which they perceive their situation. As there are so few studies of cancer patients, two models suggested in the research, on the population at large, are referred to because the same mechanisms may be effective for cancer patients. Michalos (1985) constructed a model, based on an extensive review of the literature, in which he called personal factors related to satisfaction with life as a whole, "conditioners". As can be seen from his theory, biographical variables such as age, sex, education and income are related to the evaluation of life as a whole. High self-esteem and the presence of a good social support system will also enhance the quality of life. This may also be true for cancer patients. Patients who receive positive support from their social network may be more capable of enduring the burden placed on them by the disease. Also, patients with higher self-esteem may be better able to face their situation. This is in fact what we know already from clinical practice.

Another model has been suggested by Abbey and Andrews (1985). They looked at the problem from a social psychological point of view. In their causal model, based on a large scale longitudinal study, the experience of internal control, of performance in personal life and social support predict, independent from the experience of life stress, a part of the variance of the assessment of life quality. Although the stress of life is related to the quality of life as a whole, other factors are softening this effect.

CONCLUSIONS

As has been stressed the concept of quality of life has often been used without defining it explicitly. It is suggested here that quality of life is the subjective evaluation of life as a whole. Also, the diagnosis of cancer and the process of getting through the disease experience is influenced by personal characteristics. The way cancer is dealt with is influenced by the individual's coping responses.

One may ask, what is the relevance of these theoretical points. However, they are relevant for several reasons. The variability between patients must be known in order to be able to study the impact of disease and treatment. The investigation of treatment is important when deciding upon an adequate form of therapy. The way in which people cope with a distressing situation may disguise the true effect of intrusive treatment modalities. This means that when investigating the effects of physical treatments some account must be taken of individual differences in coping response.

Moreover, by having insight into the processes by which people experience their situation it is, as Mettlin *et al.* (1983) suggested, possible to identify patients who need more support. For those who do not have a support system or a good sense of internal control over their life, or an adequate self esteem, more psychosocial care may be necessary and counselling services should be provided. In the end you might think, that more complications than solutions have been put forward so far. However, as one of my former colleagues used to say: "Life is complicated, so why should we think that the quality of life is simple?".

ACKNOWLEDGEMENTS

The author would like to thank E. Collette and F.C.E. van Knippenberg for their critical comments on an earlier version of this paper. This work was funded by the Dutch Cancer Foundation "Koningin Wilhelmina Fonds".

REFERENCES

Abbey, A. and Andrews, F. M. (1985) Modeling the psychological determinants of life quality. *Soc. Indicators Res.* **16**, 1–34.

Andrews, F. M. and Withey, S. B. (1976) *Social Indicators of Well-being.* Plenum Press, New York.

Bakker, W., Nijhuis-Heddes, J. M. A., Oosterom, A. T. van Noodijk, E. N., Hermans, J. and Dijkman, J. H. (1984) Combined modality treatment of short duration in small cell lung cancer. *Eur. J. Cancer Clin. Oncol.* **20**, 1033–1037.

Bardelli, D. and Saracci, R. (1978) Measuring the quality of life in cancer therapeutic clinical trials. *UICC Tech. Rep. Ser.* **36**, 75–97.

Borne, H. W. van den and Pruyn, J. F. A. (1985) *Lotgenoten contact bij kankerpatiënten.* Van Gorcum, Assen.

Brinkley, D. (1985) Quality of life in cancer trials. *Brit. Med. J.*. **291**, 685–686.

Bush, R. S. (1979) *Malignancies of the Ovary, Uterus and Cervix.* Edward Arnold, London.

Calman, K. (1984) Quality of life in cancer patients. *J. Med. Ethics* **10**, 125–129.

Campbell, A., Converse, P. E. and Rodgers, W. L. (1976) *The Quality of American Life.* Sage, New York.

Coates, A., Abraham, S., Kaye, S. B., Sowerbutts, T., Frewin, C., Fox, R. M., Tattersall, M. H. N. (1983) On the receiving end – patient perception of the side effects of cancer chemotherapy, *Eur. J. Cancer Clin. Oncol.*, **19**, 203–208.

70   J. C. J. M. De Haes

Doorn, C. van, Zeldenrust, M. and Asselbergs, P. (1983) Confrontatie en toekomstperspectief III. Instituut voor psychologisch marktonderzoek, Rotterdam.
Groot, A. D. de (1978) Bevordering van welzijn. In: Baerends, G. P., Groen, J. J. and de Groot, A. D. Over welzijn, Van Lochem Slaterus, Deventer.
Haes, J. C. J. M. de, Pruyn, J. F. A. and Knippenberg, F. C. E. van (1983) Klachtenlijst voor kankerpatiënten, eerste ervaringen. Ned. Tijdschr. Psych. 38, 403–422.
Haes, J. C. J. M. de and Knippenberg, F. C. E. van. (1985) The quality of life of cancer patients, a review of the literature. Soc. Sci. Med. 20, 809–817.
Haes, J. C. J. M. de, Oostrom, M. A. van and Welvaart, K. (1986) The effect of radical and conserving surgery on the quality of life of early breast cancer patients. Eur. J. Surg. Oncol. 12, 337–342.
Helson, H. and Bevan W, (1967) Contemporary Approaches to Psychology. Van Nostrand, Princeton.
Hörnquist, J. O. (1982) The concept of quality of life. Scand. J. Soc. Med. 10, 57–61.
Mettlin, C., Cookfair, D. L., Lane, W. and Pickren, J. (1983) The quality of life in patients with cancer. N.Y.Sale J. Med. febr. 187–193.
Meyerowitz, B. E., Watkins, I. K. and Sparks, F. C. (1983) Quality of life for breast cancer patients receiving adjuvant chemotherapy. Am. J. Nurs. 2, 232–235.
Michalos, A. C. (1985) Multiple discrepancies theory (MDT). Soc Indicators Res. 16, 347–413.
Michalos, A. C. (1980) Satisfaction and Happiness Soc. Indicators Res. 8, 385–422.
Padilla, G. V., Presant, C., Grant, M. M., Metter, G., Lipsett, J. and Heide, F. (1983) Quality of life index for patients with cancer. Res. Health 6, 117–126.
Priestman, T. J. and Baum, M. (1976) Evaluation of quality of life in patients receiving treatment for advanced breast cancer. Lancet 24, 899–900.
Pruyn, J. F. A. (1983) Coping with stress in cancer patients. Patient Educa. Counsel. 5, 57–62.
Schipper, H., Clinch, J., McMurray, A. and Levitt, M. (1984) Measuring the quality of life of cancer patients: the functional living index–cancer; development and validation. J. Clin. Onc. 2, 472–483.
Selby, P. J., Chapman, J. A. W., Etazadi-Amozi. J., Dalley, D. and Boyd, N. F. (1984) The development of a method for assessing the quality of life of cancer patients. Br. J. Cancer 50, 13–22.
Spitzer, W. D., Dobson, A. J., Hall, J., Chesterman, E., Levi, J., Shepherd, R., Battista, R. N. and Catchlove, B. R. (1981) Measuring the quality of life of cancer patients. A concise QL-index for use by physicians. J. Chron. Dis. 34, 585–597.
Szalaï, A. (1980) The meaning of comparative research on the quality of life. In: Szalaï, A. and Andrews, F.M. eds. The Quality of Life, Comparative Studies. Sage, London.
Weinstein, M. C. and Fineberg, H.V. (1980) Clinical Decision Analysis. W. B. Saunders, Philadelphia.
Wortman, C. B. (1984) Social support and the cancer patient: conceptual and methodological issues. Cancer 53, (10), 2339-2360.
Yalom, I. D. (1980) Existential Psychotherapy. Basic Books, New York.

Breast Self Examination and Presentation of Symptoms: Some Findings and Problems

R. GLYNN OWENS

ABSTRACT

A study by the author into factors affecting breast self-examination and promptness of presentation is used to illustrate some of the difficulties of work in this field. Although significant results were obtained, it is argued that this, and other studies in the literature, still encounter a number of problems. These are discussed under the general headings of subject, independent variable, and dependent variable problems, together with some suggestions as to how they may be overcome. The purpose of the present paper is thus not to discredit the original study but to illustrate the path for future work.

The use of screening programmes to detect early breast cancer is widely accepted as being of value in improving the prognosis of a substantial number of patients. Such screening does not, however, eliminate the need for women to perform their own screening by the use of Breast Self-Examination (BSE) procedures. Apart from questions which have been raised regarding the desirability of frequent screening and the relative precision of different techniques, it is clear that the sheer magnitude of the problem precludes the provision of facilities for all women at risk. Indeed it is arguable that the risk factors identified to date provide little help in separating out high and low risk groups for screening. Discriminant function procedures have reported only limited success in identifying groups at risk (Farewell, 1977) and at least one reviewer has concluded that ". . . at present there is no indication that high risk can be used for selective screening" (Chamberlain, 1982). BSE, therefore seems likely to have a continued role in the early detection and treatment of breast cancer.

Research into the adoption and effectiveness of BSE has generally produced disappointing conclusions. Take up rates are reported as consistently low, and little or no relationship may be found between use of BSE and outcome (Philip et al., 1984). Such results could be interpreted as suggesting that effective BSE is impractical, but other evidence (e.g. Huguley and Brown, 1981) argues against this. It is, however, becoming increasingly clear that effective BSE campaigns may need to be

71

combined with additional campaigns aimed at promptness of presentation of any symptom discovered; there is little point in detecting a symptom early if presentation of the symptom for treatment is delayed. Studies of BSE effectiveness need therefore to be considered in the context of the promptness or otherwise of the patients concerned. A corollary of this is that there is a need for effective research into the causes of patient delay. Studies in this area have been conducted for some years now, providing a wealth of (sometimes conflicting) information. It is important, however, in considering such studies, to note a number of methodological and interpretive problems. The purpose of the present paper is to illustrate a selection of such problems in the context of a typical study.

A typical study

A recent paper on women's responses to detection of breast lumps (Owens et al., 1985) may be used to illustrate some of the methodological pitfalls of research on this topic. The paper is chosen not because it is notably worse than other studies in the field, but simply because it is one with which the present author is personally involved; not only is it more honest to choose one's own work for criticism, there is also the advantage of familiarity with the material. Whilst a detailed account of the study has appeared elsewhere, the main characteristics may be summarized below.

A total of 53 first time attenders at a Liverpool breast clinic were asked to take part in the study with 50 (94%) agreeing. By means of structured interview, data were gathered on a number of dimensions including demographic factors, use of BSE, promptness of presentation and knowledge of breast cancer. Results showed that (a) 18% of the women delayed over 3 months before presenting (b) there was no relationship between use of BSE and promptness (c) knowledge was significantly correlated with promptness and (d) there was no relationship between promptness and age, parity, marital status or social class.

Like much similar research in the areas, the above study showed some consistencies and some inconsistencies with other research. Various studies report delay in presentation by around 15–25% of women (Goldstein et al., 1957; Cameron and Hinton, 1968; Philip et al., 1985). Lack of association between BSE and promptness was also noted by Philip et al. (1985), and the value of increasing knowledge of cancer has been remarked upon elsewhere (Aitken-Swann and Paterson, 1959). However the relationship of demographic factors to delay has been variously reported. Various authors have reported conflicting findings regarding the relationship between delay and such factors as marital status, age, and social class (Williams et al., 1959). Such inconsistencies hint at the role of methodological and interpretive problems in these and similar studies. Such problems may usefully be considered under the headings of subject problems, independent variable problems and dependent variable problems.

SUBJECT PROBLEMS

(a) Sample size

Whilst the total sample size of the study appears reasonable, it is still, arguably, inadequate for certain purposes. Of especial importance here is the relationship between sample size and sensitivity. In behavioural research, the dependent variable of interest is often a function of several factors, any one of which considered alone may have only a weak effect. Detection of such effects may be unreliable when sample sizes are limited. Failure to detect a relationship does not therefore permit the conclusion that no such relationship exists, but simply that none has, in this case, been found.

(b) Subgroup size

The above problem is exacerbated when the need arises to divide the sample into subgroups. In the present study of 50 women, for example, a substantial proportion (18%) delayed over 3 months: yet such a proportion reflects only nine women, a subsample size which is obviously too small to be of any great value. Similarly small numbers are apparent when other subsamples are considered (e.g. differing frequencies of BSE).

(c) Sample representativeness

It is also important to consider the extent to which any given sample adequately represents the population to whom generalization is to be made. A truly representative sample will in most cases be impractical; more usually it will be the case that the sample is determined by external factors, leaving the experimenter to determine the extent to which results may be generalized. At first glance the present sample, using 94% of those approached, might appear reasonable, although even the remaining 6% constitutes a large number when extended to the population at large. There are however additional limitations on the generalizability of the findings. The sample was, for example, limited to pre-menopausal women who had not had a hysterectomy. All the patients were attending an NHS clinic; possibly different results might have been obtained with private patients. The list of limitations could be extended, but clearly the sample is less representative than might have been hoped.

Sample problems do not permit of any totally satisfactory solution. The most obvious approach to dealing with such problems is that of increasing the total sample size. Taken alone, however, this may be an inadequate strategy, careful sample specification also being important. Researchers need to be clear, before undertaking a project, exactly which groups and subgroups need to be studied. Without such specification even a massive original sample may lead to an inadequate subsample. As an example, Philip et al.'s (1984) report of the Department of Health National Trial had an initial cohort of 22,484 women, but from this only 148 actual breast cancer patients were obtained, and only 22 women who delayed over 3 months.

Of course it is not always possible to obtain large sample sizes even when the sample characteristics are carefully identified beforehand. Thus Watson et al.'s (1984) study of women's responses to a diagnosis of breast cancer reported on only 24 such women; examination of their procedure suggests that a massive sample would have required an unrealistic time commitment. Here an attempt was made to increase sensitivity of the study by the adoption of statistical procedures, with for example significance levels of less than 0.1 being reported by contrast with more traditional levels of 0.01 or 0.05. Such a strategy increases the sensitivity of the procedure and decreases the probability of a statistical type II error (erroneous failure to reject the null hypothesis) but unfortunately at the cost of increased probability of a type I error (erroneous rejection of the null hypothesis). The trade-off between these two types of error may be a matter for the personal decision of individual researchers, although it seems likely that most will continue to use traditional significance levels.

INDEPENDENT VARIABLE PROBLEMS

Besides the problems of sample characteristics (though not entirely independent of them) are the problems of independent variables. In the study originally described it was noted that factors such as age, parity, marital status and social class failed to relate to promptness. Yet it is important to remember that the consideration of such variables will be limited by a number of factors, in particular (again) sample size. In considering the role of social class, for example, the only measure available was an initial allocation to one of the Registrar-General's classifications 1-5 on the basis of own/partner's occupation, with an approximate median split into groups 1-3a and 3b-5. Any attempt at more detailed classification would have been impractical because of the small numbers involved. Yet such a categorization is acutely insensitive to certain types of relationship, particularly those where the underlying regression is curvilinear. As an aside it is worth noting that such an analysis may also, in some instances, be effectively "hypersensitive", with an apparent relationship being suggested on the basis of only a few extreme outliers amongst the data. Once again, therefore, it is apparent that much of the inconsistency of published research may reflect nothing more than procedural variations or minor random fluctuations in a few data points. Whilst the solution to some of these problems may be straightforward (e.g. the use of transforms on skewed data, inspection for curvilinear relationships and/or the use again, of liberal significance levels) it seems likely that the greatest contribution to resolving the problem will come by the use of large, well-specified samples.

A similar problem is apparent when the adequacy of operationalizing of specific variables is considered. In considering the role of "knowledge of breast cancer", for example, it is legitimate to ask whether the link between knowledge and promptness is a continuous relationship such that the more knowledge a person has the more prompt she is likely to be, or a discontinuous one, such that the person with more knowledge in general is also more likely to have some critical item of knowledge which produces prompt presentation.

DEPENDENT VARIABLE PROBLEMS

Finally it is worth remembering that in studies in this area the dependent variables are rarely beyond question. Self-reports by patients on such data as BSE frequency, delay of presentation and the like are potentially open to several sources of error or distortion. Beside the random error likely to apply to all data collection procedures, the information obtained is likely to be subject to a number of systematic errors. Perhaps most obvious here is the risk of social desirability effects, leading to, for example, better reports of BSE use than are actually the case, or reports of more prompt presentation. Social desirability effects and other sources of error are likely, moreover, to be independent of the data. The magnitude of error involved is likely to be correlated with the interval being recalled when presentation, for example, is being considered. Thus prompt presenters may give data which is subject to proportionally more errors than delayers. Such considerations may point to the need for systematic investigations into the psychometric properties of the data, with careful consideration of their generalizability (Cronbach *et al.*, 1972). Such studies could include repeated-measures procedures, the use of between-interviewer reliability estimates and so on, and may be urgently needed if appropriate interpretation of the data is to be made.

SUMMARY AND CONCLUSIONS

It can be seen that consideration of the results of studies of BSE and delay are subject to a number of methodological and interpretive problems.

Many of these problems will occur in other areas of psychosocial oncology. At the very least there is an acute need for substantial studies to clarify the suggestive data arising from smaller studies. In particular, the status of conflicting results could be subject to close investigation. Size of sample is not however sufficient; it is important that the essential sample characteristics be specified at an early stage of the research, with particular attention being paid to the eventual size of specific subgroups and to the operationalization and analysis of independent variables. Dependent variables, too, need not necessarily be accepted at face value, and a thorough investigation is needed of the psychometric properties of measures generally taken. To answer all of these questions in a single large study is probably impractical, but if different researchers could closely coordinate their individual efforts, it seems likely that considerable progress could be made.

REFERENCES

Aitken-Swan, J. and Paterson, R. (1959) Assessment of the results of five years of cancer education. Br. Med. J. 1, 708–712.
Cameron, A. and Hinton, J. (1968) Delay in seeking treatment for mammary tumours. Cancer 21, 1121–1126.
Chamberlain, J. (1982) Screening and natural history of breast cancer. Clin. Oncol. 1, 679–701.
Cronbach, L. J., Gleser, G. C., Nanda, H. and Rajaratnam, N. (1972) The Dependability of Behavioral Measurements. John Wiley, New York.
Farewell, V. T. (1977) The combined effect of breast cancer risk factors. Cancer 40, 931–936.
Goldsen, R. K., Gerhardt, P. R., and Handy, V. H. (1957) Some factors related to patient delay in seeking diagnosis for cancer symptoms. Cancer 10, 1–7.
Henderson, J. G., Wittkower, E. D. and Lougheed, M. N. (1959) A psychiatric investigation of the delay factor in patient to doctor presentation in cancer. J. Psychosom. Res. 3, 27–41.
Huguley, C. M. Jr. and Brown, R. L. (1984) The value of breast examination. Cancer 47, 989–995.
Owens, R. G., Duffy, J. E. and Ashcroft, J. J. (1985) Women's responses to detection of breast lumps: a British study. Health Educ. J. 44, 69–70.
Philip, J., Harris, W. G., Flaherty, C., Joslin, C. A. F., Rustage, J. H. and Wijesinghe, D. P. (1984) Breast self-examination: clinical results from a population based prospective study. Br. J. Cancer, 50, 7–12.
Watson, M., Greer, S., Blake, and Shrapnell, K. (1984) Reaction to a diagnosis of breast cancer. Cancer 53, 2008–2012.
Williams, G. M., Baum, M. and Hughes, L. E. (1976) Delay in presentation of women with breast disease. Clini. Oncol. 2, 327–331.

The Interdisciplinary Treatment of Cancer: Cooperation or Competition?

LAWRENCE GOLDIE

ABSTRACT

Various forms of communication in a general hospital will be described. Particular emphasis will be upon the way in which explicit, implicit, and non-verbal forms of communication affect the relationships that exist between various professional groups and particularly between doctors. It is suggested that the modes of communication are unwittingly designed to pass on information to others whilst at the same time excluding others who are not in the group. This use of communication to include as well as exclude will be discussed in so far as it affects the transmission of the truth between professionals; the way in which it affects the freedom of the individual; and the corrupting effect that it can have on the character of the professional by reducing sensitivity and compassion.

The inter-disciplinary treatment of cancer highlights two ways in which individuals can work with one another. There is the apparent but not real co-operation when the group really has the character and nature of a "gang". The relationships in a gang are of a political nature. The individuals dissemble friendship and collude with one another in order to preserve themselves or to gain ascendancy over their companions. The other form of group is rarer and is concerned with an appreciation of the truth. Each individual is selfless and more concerned with the care of others than with the self.

My intention in this paper is to illustrate how our training inculcates and encourages the gang-like competitive group formation and that this leads to an increase rather than a decrease in suffering with a deterioration in the medical professionals' ability to cope with and endure the battlefield-type experience which is involved in dealing with cancer, the disorganization it produces, and the painful and very difficult treatments it involves.

Communication may pass on information from one group to another, but it is also used to exclude, and this can be done by the use of jargon. This was the thesis of Steiner (1975) when he discussed the reasons for the proliferation of different languages, and concluded that the group or family developed their own language so that they are understood by other members of the group; but at the same time they exclude other groups and members of other families. We know that this certainly occurs when doctors and other professionals are talking amongst themselves and unwittingly wish to maintain this separation between the medical professional and the patient, but it also plays a crucial part in maintaining and effecting a separation between different groups towards, for example, different specialists and between different professional groups such as nurses, physiotherapists and occupational therapists. As will be indicated later this is a very important source of acrimony and a lack of co-operation between groups, to the detriment of the patient. In passing one might say that whenever jargon begins to proliferate there is a proportional increase in danger for the people using it and for the people that they are caring for.

The wife of a young couple asked me one day, with a mischievous look at one another, if she had cancer; I laughed with them; it was so preposterous; she had cancer of the spine and the word had been used freely in all our discussions and we had discussed many aspects of it and the effect that it was having on their lives, and I asked "Why?". They then said thay had counted up all the different terms that had been used by doctors in place of the word "cancer'/; the list was extensive. One might ask why this word had to be replaced in the various discussions between this patient and her doctors, ostensibly and in other circumstances it might be said that the word 'cancer' is avoided in order to protect the patient, but that could not be the case here. She and her husband used the word freely so in this instance one surmises that it was not to protect the patient, but to protect the doctor who had put himself in their shoes.

We can, therefore, distinguish between two groups amongst medical professionals in hospitals; there is the group that uses language to foster a feeling of security in themselves and to effect a separation between themselves and patients and other groups. The devices used to effect this include the use of jargon and euphemisms. By 'jargon' I mean words used by a particular group so that it becomes the 'language' of that group. The euphemisms for loaded and frightening terms contain a presumption. The presumption communicated is that the patients will be more frightened and distressed by the use of plain words than by the use of euphemisms. This is a rationalization and an attempt to justify the manoeuvre. The real reason for the use of euphemisms is to protect the user. In the case notes on a ward called the "Terminal Ward" there used to be a sheet which told the nurse what the patient had been told by the surgeon or physician. The nurse was supposed to go along with the story and with the pretence. As one nurse said at the time try telling a young man whom you bath every day in potassium permanganate solution that there is nothing wrong — when the "nothing" is agonizing and his body is increasingly covered with malignant melanomata that look like weeping anuses! When I saw a physician visit this ward he was followed by a lady saying "but I'm getting worse doctor!" — he kept on walking saying briskly "Don't worry my dear — just rheumatism — it'll get better!". I do not need to elaborate upon the message *he* communicated to his companions, the nurses, the physiotherapist, and the greater audience of patients. Ultimately this type of group may be termed "self-centred" as it is for the protection of its own members. If it is a group of medical professionals one might wonder what such a group intends to protect itself from; the other groups?; patients? This kind of group I call a 'gang', because to a greater or lesser degree it has all the hallmarks of an adolescent gang. In the long run it is destructive with a prime interest in maintaining itself, which runs counter to the main function of the hospital which is to be full of care and concern *for others*. I would distinguish the "gang" from another type of group which I term a "co-operative" group. The aim of such a group is the preservation and care of others without counting the cost for the individuals in the group. The group is united by its willingness to suffer and sacrifice for others with no regard for considerations of group, class or status. As the aim of communication in the co-operative group is to pass on information which may be helpful and constructive there are no limitations and restrictions on the terms and language used. Whenever language is used the intention is the same and if any communication is unclear then efforts will be made to clarify and improve the quality of the intercourse. Improved communications result, isolating verbal screens are removed and there is increased freedom of speech between different professional practitioners.

At a recent Conference a paper was given by a nurse on the psychological care of patients, in this instance it was to a special group discussing renal dialysis. During the discussion that ensued she said that the kind of care that she was describing could not be given by doctors, only nurses could do it! When pressed she said that she did not think that doctors would understand! That communication tells us quite a lot about that nurse's view of doctors. Doctors might respond by saying that they give a different type of care with their medicine and surgery. In fact both sides are committing the same error in thinking that there is a special form of care be it "psychological" care or "medical" care. This proliferation of different groups, counsellors, specialist nurses, arises from the failure to realize that there is only one sort of care and it is either good or bad. I think this also applies to terms such as "terminal care" as if there is a special care for people who are "terminal" when in truth we are "terminal" from birth and there is still only good care. It is not the monopoly of any particular group, place or religion — though the rhetoric and propaganda of some groups try to indicate that it is. One of the difficulties of communication between different groups, for example, between nurses and doctors, is that they see the patient from different points of view, or more accurately from different worlds and the need for translating from one to the other is not realized. The nurse who bathes the young woman of her own age sees her on bedpans, stays with her to commiserate after the brief round and the devastating cursory few words that took away illusions and hope with the diagnosis; she enters into and becomes part of the patient's world. The problem is how to reduce in this instance separation between doctors and nurses so that the former appreciate the other view point and can allow themselves to know more intimately the suffering of the staff/"patient" world (they are interchangeable) and still continue to be useful to them. This may seem obvious but doctors and nurses and other medical professionals who have been ill themselves know that prior to their own, or a relative's, illness they had not by any means fully appreciated the impact of disease, hospitalization and treatment on banal, ordinary, everyday life — like a private Hiroshima. How are we to change this and to improve the communication between those who really do know and those who think they know? At the same time sensitive and compassionate medical professionals do need their breaks and a return to their private worlds where there is no sickness. This cannot be contrived, and contrary to what has been thought it cannot be produced by the formal discipline or rule book of a quasi military organization; people just cannot switch themselves on and off. The problem is, therefore, how do we produce a doctor or a medical professional who is capable of alternating between the sick patients' world and the 'healthy' world without having consciously and deliberately to *act*; to act as if the weal and woe of those who need our hospital is appreciated but instead care for and about them, naturally and without fear.

The training of medical students whilst not including training in interviewing does include training in insensitivity. Medical undergraduate training is generally by clinicians and scientists who are not only without training in teaching (a problem which has resulted in the setting up of special groups for the study of ways of improving university teaching) but are, themselves, the victims of traditional medical teaching. Most, but not all continue to use jargon and a medical history-taking procedure which eliminates from consideration the sensitive suffering individual human being. The secret language, jargon laced with euphemisms, between superiors pitying the poor (inferior) patient makes true intercourse between equals impossible. In the army, individual 'men', soldiers, became 'personnel'. 'Personnel' then perform in non-human ways — instead of washing they go to "ablutions"; they do not walk they 'proceed'. As 'personnel' they do not produce the same difficulties as 'fathers', 'brothers', 'sons', 'husbands' objects of love for wives, sisters, mothers and children. In medicine the latter become 'patients', 'cases', "the tumour on the left second bed down', 'the terminal patient', 'the geriatric problem' — thus avoiding the pain and the need to consider the unease of the whole person and his family which results from a devastating shock, similar to an unexpected explosion, which is caused by the news of the disease and its treatment. The study of physical disorder trains the student in the classification of symptoms and signs into patterns of disease, thus bringing the patient under the dissecting method, designed to isolate the disease process. As in qualitative chemical analysis the procedure is to break down the whole into its parts, in order to identify the elements of a compound.

To improve the communication between professionals in hospital regarding their charges one has to consider the meetings with patients, in any circumstances, as a privilege and an opportunity for a kind of research. I am reminded of this because I am trained and have experience as a doctor doing surgery and medicine, which I now contrast with my work as a psychotherapist or psycho-analyst, where I see patients in quite a different way. I may see, over several hours, a different patient each hour and I am making the change from one patient to another having listened carefully and responded with great deliberation to each individual. One tries, and for the most part, manages, to stop an interview and with equal sincerity and application change to accept the world of another patient. This change is not consciously made; I do not say to myself I must switch off one mood and switch on to another mood. I think this change can occur because one is doing research with each patient; following very carefully the patient and their thinking, like a research worker not leading, but following the truth wherever and whatever it may indicate. This is in contradistinction to a medical consultation in which a patient follows what is advised or described. As a doctor I already have a pattern of disease in my mind which I apply and as a doctor I am not open to receive freely and without pre-conditions what the patient has to express. My interview may be quite restricted by the questions I ask; disease and not the patient becomes the object, which is more in the nature of invention than research (Gabor, 1960). In invention the objective is known and all that might distract or deviate one from that objective is discarded. Having decided that one is to sit with another person for approximately an hour you communicate to the other person non-verbally, by the way you settle and listen, your willingness to give them the time of your life whatever their condition. They respond to this quite differently from how they may respond during 'normal' consultations in out-patients or on the ward. Referring back to the couple that I mentioned earlier who had made a list of alternative words for 'cancer'; when I first met them the patient was agonized by pain which was increased by any movement; when I sat down with her and her husband in this fashion, very tentatively but with increasing openness, they told me that they had only recently got married but they were terrified of having intercourse for fear of breaking bones in the part of the spine involved. I asked a silly question, and said had they not discussed this with the consultant or his medical team, and she laughed and said how could they possibly bring it up on a ward round, which was her only contact with the consultant, when it lasted no more than 3 minutes at her bedside. It was a public affair with the consultant's retinue around the bedside looking down at her as a specimen to be studied. Without words, this expresses for the benefit of doctors, the nursing staff and other professionals that happen to be present, what the 'chief' thinks is important and the relative value of his time compared to that of the patient. It also conveys his feelings about the value of privacy for patients and the relative value of his time compared to theirs. Memories of patients in the two contexts, medical as opposed to analytical, are quite different. Memories of people that have been seen in psychotherapy are rich and distinctive and do not depart, being akin to the memories that we are all aware of after very vivid and moving experiences of exceptional people. The recall is effortless, whereas the recall of other experiences such as routine physical examinations and the exchanges that occur in the normal medical out-patient routine require effort. This is the reason for some of the difficulties in communication between professionals. Many medical auxiliaries have dramatic and outstanding experiences with patients which they cannot forget, whereas many of their doctor colleagues have more superficial experiences, which we know to our cost they can very easily forget. Hence one is often aware of an under-current of ill-will and acrimony separating different medical professionals in hospitals, and also between different levels in a particular department. The formation of 'gangs' results in professionals being unable to speak openly to one another, having forgotten that their main concern is the patient. All too easily matters of protocol and face saving manoeuvres can over-ride consideration for the patient.

There are other important difficulties that arise because of the lack of communication between professionals who feel themselves to be at different levels. One of the reasons for this is that although there are no explicit regulations which have to be followed there is in effect a military-type organization, with ranks related to responsibility. In military-type organizations and situations, for instance, the captain of a ship, or the pilot of an aircraft appears to have total responsibility for his crew, but it is to be noted that the crew absolve themselves from responsibility; indeed they may encourage whomsoever appears to be strong and willing to accept responsibility. Obviously the communication that occurs between captains is going to be different from that which occurs between those who feel that they are without executive power. The latter may suggest, criticize and comment very carefully but may take no responsibility for what transpires. A medical registrar was reprimanded because his letter of referral stated that though the patient had cancer and was in excruciating pain, morphia which relieved the pain had been stopped because it was believed that the patient might become addicted! Apart from this being fallacious the question of addiction, even if it occurred, was not important in these circumstances. At a later date when he had left the hospital for another appointment, he made a special effort to contact the psychotherapist to tell him that, though he entirely agreed with the criticism, his "chief" at that time was convinced that morphia was addictive and he, therefore, had no option but to comply. It was perhaps courageous to admit this but erroneous in that he did have an option. It became obvious in the ensuing discussion that if it had been his father, son, or brother he would have exercised that option. He could have risked a poor reference or the loss of his job and he could have made a decision to attend to the patient's needs as he saw them. To have one set of rules for relatives and self and another for "patients" would be immoral. This form of communication may be termed an "as if" communication; over and over again one hears in hospital these "as if" communications by all levels of staff following a lapse or lack of care; it is aimed to absolve the speaker from guilt and responsibility. Knowing the truth yet speaking "as if" everyone agrees they had no option. The plea that there is no alternative but to follow instructions is inadmissible in any context. Soviet psychiatric hospitals or NHS hospitals are no different in this respect. We need to be reminded that we have the means by which we can communicate either verbally or non-verbally in hospital and show our respect for patients and their difficulties. There are non-verbal ways of communicating this; quite simply this might be done by the meticulousness with which appointments are kept; by the confidentiality exercised in transactions about patients. When we make it possible for patients to speak privately and frankly we indicate to those outside the room how much we respect the freedom of the individual even if they are ill and have limited power in the healthy world.

To instruct students of all kinds, beginners in psychotherapy, we require a different kind of teaching from traditional didactic methods. *Paris passu* with the "rational", physical, clinical, medical approach there needs to be instruction of a different kind on the same lines as used for psychotherapy training. Students would have to conduct interviews and subsequently relate them in detail with his own feelings to an experienced senior colleague. This form of supervision would be private, individual and critical. The individual would then feel that he is the instrument, here being scrutinized, to establish and maintain it at its optimum. There would in addition be presentations of individual transactions to small groups of students, with an experienced psychotherapist as supervisor. This may introduce difficulties, as some students who never want to be clinicians talking to patients may find the exposure difficult. But it would at least ensure that individuals that are very unlikely to be capable of interviewing patients would be exposed and forewarned. Some may eliminate themselves from the course — others may never interview but still have a knowledge of the problems, which enables them to support and foster the work of those that do "interview" and work by psychological means. Arranging to give private, intimate, uninterrupted time to another regardless of their state, or position relative to others in any environment requires effort to make it administratively possible, but in a hospital it is particularly difficult. To make the effort despite the seductively easy ways of avoiding the issue requires a lot of convictions about the work of human beings and a willingness to pay for this by giving to another a small part of one's life.

The principle of Complementarity orginated by Neils Bohr in Physics (1934, 1958), may be applied to under-graduate medical teaching. The medical model of disease and the non-medical model of the mind and the whole person, being complementary are not to be contrasted or compared, as commonly happens. In undergraduate teaching generally, the physical model of the non-materialistic, non-physical view of the mind is advocated. In order to introduce the psychotherapeutic approach, resistance to it would have to be explained and removed. Instead of propounding neat theories about people, encapsulated in aphorisms and generalizations, one would aim to encourage students to free themselves from prejudice and to think dynamically and flexibly in both modes at the same time. It is not necessary to reject one in order to think of the other. As in physics, the viewpoint of the observer alters the phenomena observed. Quanta and wave motion theories of light are complementary though different and incompatible — but the phenomena can be observed from either viewpoint without being contradictory. Similarly human beings can be observed from either the viewpoint of the scientist attempting to understand objective phenomena, or that of the psychoanalyst or sociologist, philosopher, psychologist attempting to understand the mind.

Encouraging the "student" however "senior" to make himself available for experiences from which he can learn is the essence of teaching. The teaching must involve discussion of interviews with patients, along with the interviewers own reactions and subjective experiences. Under the guidance of a senior experienced psychotherapist this can produce real and constructive changes in attitude. This would be in contrast to remembering facts without feelings. His position with regard to suffering could change and he would then feel that he could allow himself to think about "the hopeless case".

Traditional medical teaching includes protective devices against emotionality, and these include the use of jargon; the short time (if any) given to free and private discussions with patients; the often incredible, lack of facilities for private discussion. The short time given to patient/ doctor contact may be filled with questions and directions aimed at blocking awkward evocative responses by the patient. Physicians vary and a good physician may consciously choose to stay with the physical disease and its symptoms and leave others to consider, for example, the non-physical aspects of life such as reactions to unrelieved pain; reactions to the anticipated manner of death; and reactions to the family, social and emotional dilemmas precipitated by the disease and its treatment. Nevertheless, having had some undergraduate or post-graduate experience of psychotherapy he would know enough about what his psychotherapy colleagues attempt to do to be able to facilitate and support their efforts.

REFERENCES

Bohr, N. (1934) *Atomic Theory and the Description of Nature.* Cambridge University Press, Cambridge.
Bohr, N. (1958) *Atomic Physics and Human Knowledge.* Chapman Hall, London.
Gabor, (1960) *Inventing The Future.* Encounter, London.
Steiner, G. (1975) *After Babel. Aspects of Language and Translation.* Oxford University Press, London.

C. *Psychological Consequences*

The Psychological and Social Impact of Testicular Cancer: A Retrospective Study

CLARE MOYNIHAN, MICHAEL PECKHAM and ZARRINA KURTZ

ABSTRACT

The diagnosis and treatment of cancer is associated with substantial psychosocial morbidity, including anxiety, depression, sexual difficulties and body image problems. We wished to establish the extent of psychosocial morbidity in a sample of men with cancer of the testicle and their close relatives or friends.
We also wished to compare, retrospectively, the psychosocial outcome of men presenting with metastatic or non-metastatic disease and undergoing different treatment regimes.
Testicular cancer patients are given an excellent prognosis but despite this, we have found high levels of psychological morbidity in both the patient and the relative groups.

The psychological aspects of several types of cancer and treatment strategies have been studied extensively. Psychological and social factors have been found to influence progress of the disease once diagnosed and may make certain people more likely to develop it (Greer et al., 1979). Significant psychiatric morbidity has been found to be present in the first year after mastectomy (Greer et al., 1979; Maguire et al., 1978). Sexual maladjustment in women after mastectomy has also been shown (Maguire et al., 1978) and there is evidence of body image problems in those women who have had a breast removed (Maguire et al., 1983).

The psychological effects of surgery, radiotherapy and chemotherapy have been studied and morbidity is greater with radiotherapy or chemotherapy (Devlen, 1984; Maguire et al.,1980). It has been shown that cancer patients do not usually admit that they are experiencing problems and doctors assume that if problems have developed, patients will disclose them (Maguire et al.,1978).

We wished to examine a group of patients with cancer of the testes so that we could establish the prevalence of psychiatric and social morbidity up to 5 years following diagnosis. We also attempted to compare, retrospectively, the psychosocial outcome of men presenting with either metastic or non-metastatic disease and undergoing different

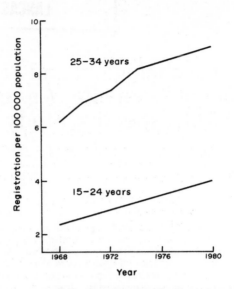

FIG. 1. REGISTRATION FOR
TESTICULAR TUMOUR PER 10 000
POPULATION IN TWO AGE GROUPS

treatment regimes. The psychosocial outcome in a close relative or friend of each patient was also studied, not only in order that we should gain a fuller understanding of the patients' situation, but because we felt that they had been largely overlooked in this area of study in Britain. Our analysis is in its preliminary stage and for the purposes of this paper, we wish to present the extent of psychological morbidity in the patients and their relative and to describe, briefly, some relevant findings that shed light on these areas.

Testicular tumours are uncommon but provide an important area for study since the incidence is rising and it is now the most common neoplasm registered among men aged between 20 and 34 (Fig. 1). During the past few years there have been major advances in clinical management, particularly the introduction of effective chemotherapy, and the cure rate is now more than 90%. Those men who do not present with evidence of metastases may now be managed by orchidectomy alone followed by close surveillance. Although approximately 20% of these relapse within the first year, subsequent chemotherapy is highly effective.

The disease strikes young men at a time of important family and career responsibilities. Although 'cured' the men have suffered the impact of diagnosis of a potentially fatal condition, the loss of a sexual organ and the toxicity of treatment including infertility which may not be

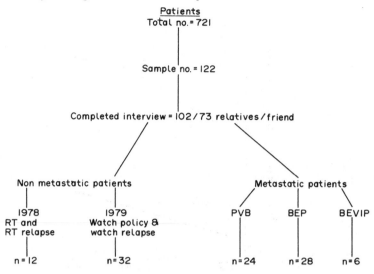

Patients
Total no. = 721

Sample no. = 122

Completed interview = 102/73 relatives/friend

Non metastatic patients

1978 RT and RT relapse	1979 Watch policy & watch relapse
n = 12	n = 32

Metastatic patients

PVB	BEP	BEVIP
n = 24	n = 28	n = 6

97 patients and 69 relatives/friend completed BOTH an interview and a present state examination

FIG. 2. STUDY DESIGN

recovered. A proportion of patients who undergo surgery for residual abdominal masses also suffer subsequent failure to ejaculate. Usually, however, normal erection and orgasm are possible.

METHOD

Patients

We randomly selected a stratified sample from 721 men who had been referred to the Royal Marsden Hospital, London and Surrey from January 1976 to December 1983. Figure 2 shows the study design. Patients treated elsewhere and all those treated prior to 1978 with outdated treatment protocols were excluded.

The remaining 540 patients were stratified according to the type of initial management, age, year of first referral and social class. The following treatment groups were selected: Radiotherapy (RT), Surveillance (W), Surveillance relapse (WR), Chemotherapy (PVB, BEP, BEVIP).

We randomly selected a total of 122 patients who were contacted by letter inviting them to an interview. Full background and aims of the study were enclosed. One hundred and two patients (84%) responded and were subsequently interviewed. For each respondent a close relative or friend was asked to participate. Seventy-three relatives

TABLE 1. STRATIFICATION OF THE SAMPLE ACCORDING TO PATIENTS' AGE, TREATMENT GROUP, YEAR OF
DIAGNOSIS AND SOCIAL CLASS

Age of patient	15–19 (n = 12)		20–24 (n = 22)		25–29 (n = 23)	30–34 (n = 18)	35–39 (n = 11)	>40 (n = 11)	Total (n = 97)
*Treatment groups	RT 4	RTR 8	W 16	WR 13	PVB 23	BEP 27	BEVIP 6		97
Year of diagnosis	78/79 n = 21		80 n = 26		81 n = 16	82 n = 17	83 n = 17		97
Social class	Non manual n = 50				Manual n = 46		Retired n = 1		97

*RT = Radiotherapy; RTR = Radiotherapy relapse; W = Watch Surveillance Group;
WR = Watch Surveillance Group who have relapsed;
PVB, BEP, BEVIP = Chemotherapy regimes

(relative = relative or friend combined) responded to our invitation and were interviewed. Ninety-seven patients and 69 relatives completed both the interview and the Present State Examination (PSE). The entry criteria (age, social class, severity of illness, type of treatment and year of entry) in patients and relatives who did not respond to the interview request were not statistically different from the studied group.

The interview

At each interview a specially designed semi-structured questionnaire was completed. A PSE (Wing *et al.*,1974) was carried out with each man and close relative. The main areas covered in both the patients' and the relatives'/friends' interview were as follows:

Demographic factors, medical history, family history, sexual history, social history (including support systems), hospital experience, patients, perceptions of aspects of his illness, relative's particular worries covering their involvement with the patient, body image.

The Present State Examination

The PSE is a standardized instrument for measuring anxiety and depression (Wing *et al.*, 1974). In this study, a person was rated as either an anxious or depressed 'case' if he or she suffered nervous tension or depression and four other related symptoms in the month prior to interview. A 'borderline' case exhibited the same main symptoms outlined above but he or she had fewer related symptoms. Intensity and frequency of symptoms were determining factors in the rating of a case.

RESULTS

Reliability

The PSE was tape recorded in order that a reliability check with an independent rater could be carried out. Agreement between the

TABLE 2. PATIENTS AND RELATIVES OR FRIENDS RATED AS
A CASE ON PSE EXAMINATION

	Patients (n = 97)	%	Relatives (n = 69)	%
Case	22	23	15	22

TABLE 3. PREVALENCE OF PATIENTS' SYMPTOMS OF ANXIETY AND
DEPRESSION BROKEN DOWN INTO CASES AND BORDERLINE CASE

	Anxiety		Depression	
	n	%	n	%
Case	11	11	5	5
Borderline	3	3	3	3
Total cases	14	14	8	8

Total number of men showing symptoms of anxiety and
depression = 22 (23%).

TABLE 4. PREVALENCE OF RELATIVES' SYMPTOMS OF ANXIETY AND
DEPRESSION BROKEN DOWN INTO CASES AND BORDERLINE CASE

	Anxiety		Depression	
	n	%	n	%
Case	7	10	3	4
Borderline	3	4	2	3
Total cases	10	14	5	7

Total number of relatives showing symptoms of anxiety and
depression = 15 (22%).

interviewer and the independent rater was high on all the main
symptoms (95% agreement, κ = 0.86, $P < 0.001$).

The proportion of patients and relatives and friends who showed
psychological morbidity is shown in Table 2. When the PSE ratings were
broken down into case and borderline cases, anxiety and depression, the
prevalence of anxiety exceeds that of depression in both the patient and
relative/friends group. Of the patients, 14% suffered symptoms of
anxiety and 8% from depression while 14% of relatives/friends suffered
symptoms of anxiety and 7% from symptoms of depression (Tables 3 and
4).

Patients' psychological morbidity and related factors

Factors examined in relation to the patients' symptoms of psychological
morbidity are shown in Table 5. Statistical significance was only found in
relation to the patient's age at time of diagnosis of his tumour. Certain
trends, however, were distinguishable and are as follows:

TABLE 5. FACTORS EXAMINED WITH RELATION
TO PSE RATINGS OF PATIENTS

Age*
Treatment types
Length of time since first referral to Royal Marsden Hospital
Marital status
Social class
Sexual problems
Body image

$$*\chi^2 = 12.95, P < 0.05$$

Age

The highest rates of morbidity were found in the youngest age group. Forty-two per cent of the very youngest (15-19 years) suffered symptoms compared to 17% of those who were aged over 30. This revealed a statistical significance of $\chi^2 = 12.9, P < 0.05$.

Treatment types

The highest levels of psychological morbidity were found in patients who had the most toxic treatment regime (BEVIP): 33%, and those who had been in the surveillance group (Watch policy) but had relapsed within a year: 33%. The levels of psychological morbidity in men who had ungergone other treatment regimes including Watch policy without relapse, although lower, were not significantly different.

Length of time since first referral

Those men who had most recently been diagnosed had the highest rate of psychological morbidity. Of those who were diagnosed in 1983, 41% were rated as a case, whereas 24% of those who entered the hospital in 1978/1979 showed symptoms of psychological disturbance. Apart from this trend, the length of time since treatment did not appear to have an effect. The proportion of psychological morbidity in men who had been diagnosed in 1978 and 1979 was marginally higher than those who entered in 1982.

Marital status and social class

The presence of psychological symptoms was independent of marital status and social class, although those who were single at diagnosis were more likely to be at psychological risk at interview.

Sexual problems

Sexual problems were reported to be uncommon before diagnosis and treatment started, although twenty five men said they had no sex life at

TABLE 6. FACTORS EXAMINED WITH RELATION
TO PSE RATINGS OF RELATIVES AND FRIENDS

Age of patient
Length of time since diagnosis*
Partners/non partners at interview
Proximity to patient during treatment
Number of children at interview†
Sperm banking
Fertility status of partner at interview

$*\chi^2 = 8.2, P<0.05$
$†\chi^2 = 4.0. P<0.05$

that time. At the time of interview, 25% of the men had noticed a deterioration in this area. This was not related to age, type of treatment and length of time since starting treatment. The proportion of men with psychological morbidity was no higher in those who reported an inability to ejaculate: only one of these was suffering from symptoms of anxiety,

Body image

At the time of interview, patients did not appear unduly worried about their body image, nor was psychological morbidity related to particular aspects of their image such as a desire for a testicular prostheses. Worry over hair loss during treatment was also found to be unrelated to symptoms of anxiety and depression at interview.

Relative/friends psychological morbidity and related factors

Factors examined in relation to the relatives/friends symptoms of psychological morbidity are shown in Table 6. Statistical significance was found in relation to the length of time since the patients' diagnosis, and the number of children at interview. Certain trends, however, were distinguishable and are as follows:

Age of patient

Psychological cases were independent of the age of the patient although there was a higher proportion of morbidity in those relative/friends whose husbands, sons or friend were in the over 30 age group.

Time since diagnosis and start of treatment of patient

Relatives/friends of patients who had been diagnosed in 1983 showed significantly higher levels of psychological morbidity ($\chi^2 = 8.2, P<0.05$). Of those relatives/friends who had been most recently subjected to the stress of diagnoses, 50% showed signs of psychological disturbance whereas of those who had had that experience in 1978/1979 only 23% showed signs of morbidity.

Number of children at interview

Wives and live-in girlfriends who were childless at interview were significantly more anxious and depressed than those who had had one or more children (x^2 = 4.0, $P < 0.05$), 38% of these partners with no children showed psychological morbidity, while 14% did so if they were parents. Psychological symptoms of the wives and live-in partners were independent of the patients' fertility status although the proportion of morbidity was higher in those whose partners were infertile, regardless of whether they had children or not. The knowledge that sperm had been banked or not, was not related to psychological morbidity in these partners.

'Live-in' relatives at the time of interview

The proportion of relatives/friends with psychological morbidity was higher if they were not living with the patient at the time of interview. Psychological morbidity was also found to be higher in those who had been living with the patient when he was undergoing treatment.

DISCUSSION

Our preliminary findings show high levels of psychological morbidity in both patients and relatives. This is confirmed when compared with a community study carried out by Dean et al. (1983) with women in Edinburgh. Using a version of the PSE, they found a rate of 9% in a representative population sample. That the rates of psychological morbidity are higher in the patient group is not surprising since similar findings have been recorded in other cancer types, especially where mutilating surgery has been carried out (Maguire, 1983; Devlin et al., 1971).

Although we were aware that relatives and friends were anxious about their loved ones, we were surprised at the significantly high levels of morbidity in this group. Data gathered at interview, which has not been the primary subject of this paper, show that in the majority of cases, despite the most caring of hospital staff, psychological morbidity and/or sexual problems had not been formally identified by clinicians and general practitioners and that this aspect of care had not been built into the framework of therapy. The patients, like their spouses, sons and friends, found it difficult to voice their anxieties outside their families and, even within them, the most intense worries were often not discussed. While the patient at least, had the advantage of pastoral care provided by family, hospital staff and the therapeutic value provided by the atmosphere created on the hospital wards, the relatives' main contribution throughout their experience appears to have been the presentation of a "brave face" – a façade which patients particularly appreciated and interpreted as "strength" and "normality". We found that the relatives expressed an overwhelming desire for formal support. This may have been a reflection of their need to talk through their anxieties.

Even though these are patients and relatives who belong to a particular cancer group, it is likely that our findings are generally applicable to others. In particular, we feel that families of sufferers should be offered formal support of some kind.

This study validates the findings that cancer patients with a good prognosis have high levels of psychological morbidity. Time, however, does not appear to be having an alleviating effect although our data shows that there was an indication that the 5 year 'magic marker' of remission may help to diminish psychological distress. Even among many of the relatives, the passage of time does not appear to have healed their anxieties.

Our findings do not suggest that the levels of psychological morbidity are particularly high in those who had radiotherapy or chemotherapy or both. This finding has wide implications. Contrary to expectations, a "wait and see" approach may be difficult to cope with, although the men had been made aware that they have been diagnosed at an early stage and that their prognosis is excellent. It also suggests that an aggressive treatment regime may, itself, have a therapeutic effect (Revenson, 1983). Many of the men in the surveillance group described the tension they had experienced as they went on waiting to be told the worst. "If I had had chemotherapy, the waiting would all be over by now." On the other hand, all patients from all treatment groups were anxious that their disease may recur. When asked what their most worrying problem was at the time of interview, recurrence appears to be the men's main preoccupation and is a similar one to that reported elsewhere (Kennedy *et al.*, 1976).

The young, unmarried men were more likely to suffer symptoms of anxiety and depression and this may possibly indicate that close ties have not been established at that particular time in the life cycle. A confiding relationship may be essential to the well-being of this group. A more in-depth analysis will enable us to make a clearer assessment as to whether this group did indeed have close ties at the time of treatment and interview. If they did not, the effects of counselling on this particular category of patient may be well worth exploring.

We were interested to find that having a child appears to make a

98   *Clare Moynihan, Michael Peckham and Zarrina Kurtz*

difference to the psychological well-being of a "live-in" partner. Interestingly, our data show that *all* relatives/friends, whether they were partners or not, show less psychological morbidity when there was a child in the family or if the possibility of having one had been confirmed. Having a child was seen not only as a naturally joyous and life-enhancing event ("it carried us through"), but was also perceived as a sign of cure. Further analysis will give us more information surrounding this very important area.

Not surprisingly, being close to the patients' experience of the consequences of treatment has an effect on the relatives but trends also suggest that those not living with the patients at interview were more prone to psychological morbidity. Further analysis will reveal whether mothers/fathers or partners predominated in either situation and whether they were more tense according to their relationship with the patient.

Body image does not appear to be a particularly worrying aspect of the men's experience. This finding was reinforced by the fact that, although testicular prostheses are available and usually offered, generally, they did not seem to be necessary to the men. However, clinicians dealing with testicular cancer patients should attempt to discuss the loss of a testicle and the profound effect it *may* have on some of them. Declarations such as "you can fly on one cylinder as well as two" may only be partly reassuring and leaves many questions unanswered.

Hair loss was seen as fashionable and therefore not necessarily stressful. This may be a shifting phenomenon, however, and as fashions change, the men's attitude towards their body image, especially during treatment may become more negative.

These preliminary findings raise a number of questions which we will address in further analysis. But even at this early stage, our findings show very clearly that men with this type of cancer, and their relatives, have problems which have sometimes been unnoticed.

REFERENCES

Dean, C., Surtees, P. G. and Sashidharan, S. P. (1983) Comparison of research diagnostic systems in and Edinburgh community sample. *Br. J. Psychiat.* **142**, 247–256.
Devlin, J. (1984) Psychosocial and social aspects of Hodgkin's disease and non-Hodgkin's lymphoma. PhD Thesis, University of London.
Devlin, B. H., Plant, J. A. and Griffin, M. (1971) Aftermath of surgery for anorectal cancer. *Br. Med. J.* **3**, 413–418.
Greer, S., Morris, T. and Pettingale, K. W. (1979) Psychological response to breast cancer: effect on outcome. *Lancet* **i**, 785–787.
Kennedy, B. J., Auke Telhegen, M. and Kennedy, S. (1976) Psychological response of patients cured of advanced cancer. *Cancer* **38**, 2184–2191.
Maguire, G. P., (1983) The psychological impact of cancer. *Br. J. Hosp. Med.* **34** (2), 100–103.

Maguire, G. P., Lee, E., Bevington, D., Cushemann, C. S., Crabtree, R. J. and Cornell, C. E. (1978) Psychiatric problems in the first year after mastectomy. *Br. Med. J.*, 963-965.

Maguire, G. P., Tait, A., Brooke, M., Thomas, C. and Sellwood, R. (1980) Effect of counselling on the psychiatric morbidity associated with mastectomy. *Br. Med. J.* 1454-1456.

Maguire, G. P., Brooke, M., Tait, Thomas, C. and Sellwood, R. (1983) The effect of counselling on physical disability and social recovery after mastectomy. *Clin. Oncol.* **9**, 319-324.

Revenson, T. A. (1983) Social supports as stress buffers for adult cancer patients. *Psychosom. Med.* **45**, 321-331.

Wing, J. K., Cooper, J. E. and Sartorious, N. (1974) *Measurement of Classification of Psychiatric Symptoms*. Cambridge University Press, Cambridge.

The Psychological Impact of Adjuvant Chemotherapy following Mastectomy

A. V. MARK HUGHSON and A. F. COOPER

ABSTRACT

Psychological symptoms were assessed over 2 years in a randomized trial of three forms of treatment following mastectomy for Stage II breast cancer. The treatments were: 3 weeks' radiotherapy; 1 year's adjuvant cyclophosphamide, methotrexate and 5-fluorouracil; radiotherapy followed by chemotherapy. Analysis of the results on an intention to treat basis showed no substantial differences in depression or anxiety among groups at 1, 3 and 6, months after operation. At 13 months, however, patients who had been allocated chemotherapy had significantly more symptoms, especially depression, than control patients who had received radiotherapy alone. Conditioned reflex nausea and vomiting increased markedly during the second 6 months of chemotherapy, and persisted for up to a year thereafter.

The psychological morbidity of adjuvant chemotherapy could be substantially reduced if courses of treatment were restricted to about 6 months.

"... I know of nothing more cruel, nothing more frightful, that the spectacle of unfortunate patients who have been operated on, and in whom the cancer has become reproduced. To see them day by day, and week by week, and not to know what to say, by what expressions to give them consolation, what drugs to recommend to give them patience, what aspect of countenance to assume, to hide them from the despair with which they are filled, is genuine martyrdom" (Velpeau, 1856).

The sorrow of the distinguished 19th century French surgeon on seeing his breast cancer patients relapse will be familiar to any sensitive doctor treating such patients today. However, there is now general agreement that adjuvant chemotherapy delays systemic relapse and death in early breast cancer. Analysis of the results of clinical trials in some 10,000 patients has shown that adjuvant chemotherapy reduces the number of early deaths in postmenopausal women by about one sixth and in premenopausal women by about one third (Anonymous, 1984). But will such treatment cause despair as well as perhaps prevent it?

A randomized trial of chemotherapy in Stage II breast cancer (McArdle et al., 1986) provided an opportunity to examine the psychological consequences of adjuvant treatment (Hughson et al., 1986).

101

A. V. Mark Hughson and A. F. Cooper

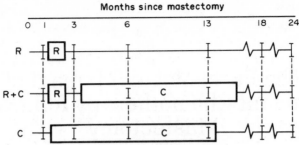

FIG. 1. DESIGN OF TRIAL SHOWING TIMING OF
PSYCHOLOGICAL ASSESSMENTS. R = RADIOTHERAPY.
C = CHEMOTHERAPY. R + C = RADIOTHERAPY PLUS
CHEMOTHERAPY. BARS REPRESENT TIMES
OF ASSESSMENTS.

PATIENTS AND METHODS

Figure 1 shows the design of the study. Consecutive patients under the age of 70 underwent simple mastectomy and were allocated at random to:

(i)   A 3 week course of radiotherapy to chest wall and local lymph nodes;

(ii)   A year of chemotherapy;

(iii)   Radiotherapy followed by chemotherapy.

The chemotherapy regime was similar to that of Bonadonna in Italy except that all drugs were given intravenously (Bonadonna *et al.*, 1976). Cyclophosphamide, methotrexate and 5-fluorouracil (CMF) was administered on an outpatient basis on days 1 and 8 of consecutive 28 day cycles.

Psychological morbidity was measured with four point observer rating scales of depression and anxiety developed by Maguire for his 1978 mastectomy study (0 absent, 1 mild, 2 moderate, 3 severe) (Maguire *et al.*, 1978). Self rating scales were also used: the Leeds General Scales for the self assessment of depression and anxiety (Snaith *et al.*, 1976) and the General Health Questionnaire (Goldberg, 1979). The Leeds scales were modified slightly to cover the same time period as the General Health Questionnaire and the observer scales, namely the few weeks preceding interview. Scores on both Leeds scales range from 0 to 18, and scores of 7 or above indicate a high probability of clinical depression or anxiety.

Scores on the General Health Questionnaire range from 0 to 60, but it contains somatic items such as lack of energy which might be endorsed by patients with purely physical distress. False positives might occur if the normal threshold score of 12 or above were taken to indicate psychological morbidity. Therefore the severe depression subscale of the General Health Questionnaire, which consists of specific psychic items such as ideas of suicide, worthlessness and hopelessness, was analysed separately. Scores on this subscale range from 0 to 21, but there is no recognized threshold score. A small validation study, using scores obtained a year after mastectomy from an earlier cohort of 44 patients participating in the same chemotherapy trial, was performed. With a Maguire depression observer rating of 2 or above as the criterion for psychological morbidity, scores of 3 or above on the severe depression subscale gave satisfactory discrimination between "cases" and "non-cases", with a sensitivity of 75% and a specificity of 89% (Six of eight "cases" and 32 of 36 "non-cases" were correctly classified.)

A simple physical symptom score was devised, based on the presence of several key symptoms in the month prior to assessment. These included anorexia, nausea, vomiting, mucosal irritation, hair loss, skin reaction, pain and dyspnoea. One point was allotted for each symptom present. The presence of conditioned reflect nausea and vomiting was noted (Neese et al., 1980).

Assessments at the times shown in Figure 1 allowed psychological and physical morbidity to be measured before treatment, following radiotherapy, midway through the course of chemotherapy, shortly before completion of chemotherapy, and 5 and 11 months after the completion of chemotherapy. Patients receiving chemotherapy were reviewed at the end of the "rest" period, as close as possible to day 28 of each cycle, and those who had completed radiotherapy were seen 2-3 weeks after treatment. Thus interviews relating to treatment were timed so as to minimize confusion between physical and psychological symptoms.

Most patients were interviewed at home by the first author. Inter-rater reliability for the two authors was checked in 16 patients. Kappa values (Cohen, 1968) for depression and anxiety were 0.74 and 0.68 respectively.

Results were analysed on an intention-to-treat basis. All patients were included regardless of whether they had relapsed or failed to complete chemotherapy. Statistical tests (two-tailed) were as follows: for comparisons among groups, χ^2 tests, Fisher exact tests and Kruskal–Wallis analysis of variance; for comparisons within groups, McNemar's χ^2 test for correlated proportions and the binomial test.

RESULTS

Seventy-four of 79 consecutive patients agreed to take part in the psychological study. The mean age of the sample was 52.4 years. The treatment groups were similar in respect of age, social class, marital status and previous psychiatric history. Similar numbers were allocated to each type of treatment (Table 1). During the study, six patients refused further psychiatric interviews and six more refused to continue

TABLE 1. NUMERS OF PATIENTS WHO REFUSED FURTHER INTERVIEWS OR FURTHER CHEMOTHERAPY, RELAPSED, OR DIED DURING STUDY

Treatment	Radiotherapy	Chemotherapy	Combined treatment
Agreed to participate	24	27	23
Refused further interviews	1	5	0
Refused further chemotherapy (but not further interviews)	—	3	3
Recurrence			
Local	0	4	0
Systemic*	10	4	2
Died	9	3	3

*A few patients who developed systemic relapse died before they could be re-interviewed.

TABLE 2. NUMBERS OF PATIENTS RECEIVING EACH TYPE OF TREATMENT DURING STUDY

Months since operation	Radiotherapy	Chemotherapy	Combined treatment
1	24	27	23
3	23	25	23
6	23	24*	23
13	21†	24*	22
18	18†	21	20
24	14	19	20

*Sample size one less for self rating scales as one patient felt too depressed to complete them.
†Sample size two less for self rating scales as patients felt too ill physically to complete them.

chemotherapy but agreed to further interviews. Systemic relapse and deaths were commoner in patients allocated radiotherapy, occurring especially in the second year after operation. More than a third of the radiotherapy patients had died by the end of the study, compared with less than a sixth in the two chemotherapy groups. Table 2 shows sample sizes at each assessment.

The prevalence of psychological morbidity measured by Maguire's scales is shown in Fig. 2. One month following mastectomy in the radiotherapy-alone group the prevalences of anxiety and depression were 33 and 38%, both falling to 14% at 1 year. The prevalence of anxiety and depression in the two chemotherapy groups was similar, at 1, 3 and 6 months. However at 13 months there was a significant excess of anxiety ($P < 0.05$) and an excess of depression ($P < 0.1$) in both chemotherapy groups. In the second year, psychological morbidity fell in the two chemotherapy groups, but at 18 months seemed to rise in radiotherapy-alone group. However, virtually all the psychological morbidity in that group occurred in five patients with systemic relapse. All five scored positively for anxiety or depression, compared with none of the disease-free survivors.

Figure 3 shows the results of the Leeds self-rating scales. The pattern is similar to that seen on the observer scales. There were no significant

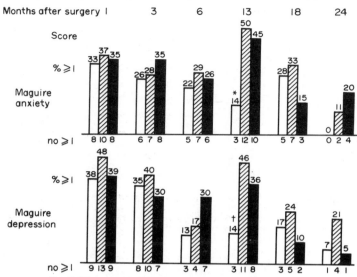

FIG. 2. MAGUIRE OBSERVER SCALES: PROPORTIONS (%) WITH
PSYCHOLOGICAL MORBIDITY. ☐ RADIOTHERAPY; ▨ CHEMOTHERAPY;
■ RADIO + CHEMOTHERAPY. *$P < 0.05$;
†$P < 0.1$ (χ^2 TESTS WITH 2° OF FREEDOM)

differences amongst groups up to 6 months, but at 13 months, both groups
allocated to chemotherapy showed an excess of psychological morbidity
compared with radiotherapy-alone controls. This excess was
statistically significant on the Leeds depression scale ($P < 0.03$). About a
quarter of patients allocated chemotherapy alone or in combination had
clinical depression as judged by the Leeds scale. In the second year less
psychological morbidity was evident.

Results of the General Health Questionnaire and severe depression
subscale (Fig. 4) resembled those of the Leeds scales. At 13 months there
was more psychological morbidity in both groups allocated to
chemotherapy. The excess was significant on the severe depression
subscale ($P < 0.03$). Again about a quarter of patients allocated
chemotherapy alone or in combination showed clinical depression.

Physical symptom scores (Table 3) were similar among groups up to 3
months after operation. At 6 and 13 months there were more physical
problems in the two chemotherapy groups, compared with the
radiotherapy-alone controls. At 18 months, this trend was reversed,
because systemic relapse was common in the radiotherapy-alone group
but not in the chemotherapy groups.

Three months after operation conditioned reflex nausea without
vomiting was present in three patients receiving chemotherapy alone
and two who had received radiotherapy alone. At 6 months in both
groups allocated to chemotherapy ($n = 47$) a third of patients had

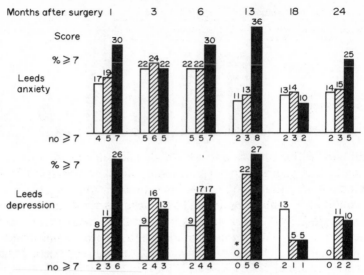

FIG. 3. LEEDS SELF-RATING SCALES: PROPORTIONS (%) WITH
PSYCHOLOGICAL MORBIDITY. *P<0.03 (USING FISHER EXACT TEST WITH
CHEMOTHERAPY AND RADIOTHERAPY PLUS CHEMOTHERAPY GROUPS
COMBINED BECAUSE OF SMALL EXPECTED FREQUENCIES)

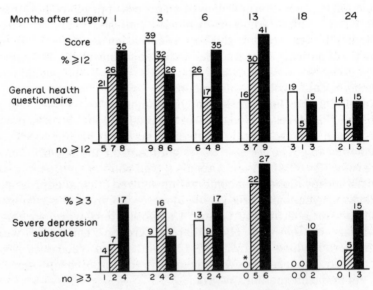

FIG. 4. GENERAL HEALTH QUESTIONNAIRE AND SEVERE DEPRESSION
SUBSCALE: PROPORTIONS (%) WITH PSYCHOLOGICAL MORBIDITY.
*P<0.03; (USING FISHER EXACT TEST WITH CHEMOTHERAPY AND
RADIOTHERAPY PLUS CHEMOTHERAPY GROUPS COMBINED BECAUSE OF
SMALL EXPECTED FREQUENCIES)

TABLE 3. MEAN SCORES FOR PHYSICAL SYMPTOMS

Months since operation	Radiotherapy	Chemotherapy	Combined treatment
1	0.2	0.2	0.3
3	3.2	3.4	3.1
6	0.4*	3.8	3.6
13	0.7*	3.7	3.8
18	1.3†	0.3	0.3
24	1.0	0.1	0.3

*$P<0.001$; †$P<0.1$ (Kruskal-Wallis test on differences among groups)

conditioned reflex nausea and 13% had conditioned reflex vomiting. By 13 months, the prevalence of conditioned reflex symptoms had virtually doubled. Of 46 patients, 59% had conditioned reflex nausea, and 35% had conditioned reflex vomiting. The increases were highly significant ($P<0.002$ and $P<0.01$ for nausea and vomiting respectively in the 46 patients alive at both assessments). Furthermore, conditioned reflex symptoms persisted beyond treatment. At 18 months 27% of 41 patients in the two groups allocated chemotherapy had conditioned reflex nausea and 7% had conditioned reflex vomiting. Even at 24 months, 18% of 39 patients still had conditioned reflex nausea.

Most often the conditioned stimulus was the sight or smell of the hospital and medical equipment such as syringes and needles, but anything associated with the nausea and vomiting caused by treatment might subsequently of itself induce the same symptoms. One woman vomited when she saw a member of the clinic staff in a shop. Other stimuli included clothes worn or perfume used whilst attending for treatment, foods cooked at home during post-treatment vomiting, or the mere thought of treatment. Where possible patients sought to avoid experiencing such stimuli again (though many forced themselves to keep clinic appointments during and after treatment, despite conditioned reflex symptoms, or were firmly escorted to the hospital by their husbands.) A year after completing treatment, a 31-year-old patient talked of her "sick coat". She had worn it during treatment, but now it was hidden at the back of her wardrobe, to stop her feeling sick again. Another patient who had completed chemotherapy tried to remove the nauseous smell of the hospital from some of her clothes by washing them repeatedly. After her attempts had failed she threw the clothes away.

At the assessment at six months patients were asked their opinions about their treatment. In the combined treatment group all but two of the 23 patients were already certain that chemotherapy was more unpleasant than radiotherapy ($P<0.001$). One patient said that chemotherapy was the worst thing that had ever been thought up. A highly competent deputy headteacher with severe conditioned reflex vomiting described the utter humiliation she felt at losing control of herself so unexpectedly, in front of everyone at the hospital. However, certain patients who had expressed hatred of chemotherapy subsequently became apprehensive when it was stopped. Regular check-ups at the clinic had reassured them, despite the unpleasantness of the actual treatment.

Hair loss did not seem a serious source of distress for most patients. Good wigs were provided. Nausea and vomiting were very distressing, even when conditioned reflex symptoms were not superimposed. A few patients reported sexual problems specific to chemotherapy. One problem was dyspareunia, presumably caused by the adverse effect of chemotherapy on epithelial surfaces, and another was anxiety about contraception. Two patients were worried they might conceive a child who would be malformed by chemotherapy.

Chemotherapy was the only treatment to induce suicidal thoughts, though these were not persistent, tending to occur when physical toxicity was maximal. They were never acted on. With the exception of one woman with a long history of endogenous depression antedating mastectomy, no patient required admission to a psychiatric ward.

It was of interest to estimate the true magnitude of the depressive effect of CMF. Both the Leeds depression scale and severe depression scale of the general health questionnaire gave virtually identical results, with around 25% of 45 patients allocated CMF alone or in combination experiencing clinical depression at 13 months (when it was intended they should complete treatment, though six of the 45 did not do so). Since an earlier cohort of patients had also been studied at 13 months, it was possible to pool data to give results for 75 such patients at 13 months. Results of the same two depression scales were again identical: both classed 28% of 75 patients intended to complete CMF (either alone or following radiotherapy) as clinically depressed. The 95% confidence intervals were 18–38%. So, in round terms, the true proportion in the population from which the sample was drawn probably lay between one fifth and one third, and would have been marginally higher had patients not completing CMF been excluded.

The virtual absence of clinical depression in radiotherapy patients at 13 months was surprising and prompted a similar look at data pooled from the present and earlier cohorts. In 34 radiotherapy-alone patients at 13 months, only one was classed depressed by the severe depression scale and two (6%) by the Leeds depression scale. Valid confidence intervals could not be calculated, however, for such low proportions.

DISCUSSION

In the past, randomized controlled studies of the psychological effects of adjuvant chemotherapy in breast cancer have tended to rely on single estimates of morbidity during treatment. Preliminary results of the present study (Hughson *et al.*,1980), and other subsequent reports from the United Kingdom (Maguire *et al.*, 1980; Palmer *et al.*, 1980) were in this category. However, all suggested that adjuvant chemotherapy—in particular cyclophosphamide, methotrexate and 5-fluorouracil (CMF) — was associated with increased emotional distress. Two studies caused doubts to be expressed as to whether such treatment could be justified (Palmer *et al.*, 1980; Howell *et al.*, 1984).

In the United States, adjuvant chemotherapy has been more widely adopted as routine treatment. Probably for that reason, quantitative studies of its psychological effects have been lacking (Consensus Conference, 1985). However, in an uncontrolled study, Meyerowitz *et al.* (1979) noted that up to 80% of breast cancer patients undergoing adjuvant treatment with CMF experienced emotional distress. Follow-up showed that quality of life was often impaired for several months beyond treatment (Meyerowitz *et al.*, 1983). A more recent uncontrolled study of similar patients also suggested that distress persisted beyond treatment (Knobf, 1986). In contrast are the early results of a study comparing self-rated anxiety levels in 68 mastectomy patients randomized to CMF plus prednisolone (CMFP), or to observation only (Cassileth *et al.*, 1986). Assessments over 1 year showed no significant differences between the two groups, but there was a trend towards higher anxiety levels in patients not given adjuvant treatment. The authors thought that allocation to observation only might induce anxiety, whilst active treatment might have a placebo effect. The results are not altogether comparable with other studies of the psychological effects of CMF, since steroids may affect mood, and levels of depression were not reported.

In the present study, several assessments over 2 years allowed a more detailed review of the psychological cost of CMF. Adjuvant chemotherapy had its main psychological impact during the second half of intended treatment. Depression and conditioned reflex symptoms peaked at 1 year, even though over a tenth of patients did not complete CMF. Conditioned reflex symptoms continued beyond the first year. Depression may also have persisted in minor degree. However, most patients allocated chemotherapy escaped systemic relapse in the second year. Unlike the radiotherapy-alone patients, they were spared much of the emotional and physical distress associated with recurrent disease.

The peak of psychological morbidity during the second half of CMF, and some of the after-effects, could almost certainly be abolished if courses of treatment were restricted to about 6 months. Since 6 months of adjuvant CMF is probably as effective as 12 (Bonadonna *et al.*, 1985), there seems little justification at present for longer courses of CMF.

Several questions remain unanswered. Whilst psychological morbidity could be substantially reduced by shortening courses of chemotherapy, it is unclear whether the lifetime psychological cost to the patient due to adjuvant chemotherapy would thereby become similar to that due to radiotherapy alone. The precise lifetime cost could only be determined by indefinite follow-up of a very large series of patients. Much would depend on the varying effects and timing of relapses, further treatments and deaths after the first 2 years. These matters are complex. Although the present study and that of Silberfarb et al., (1980) show, not surprisingly, that recurrent disease is distressing, treatment given for systemic relapse may sometimes reduce morbidity. Thus Baum et al., (1980) found that chemotherapy given for systemic relapse enhanced well-being, despite physical toxicity, provided remission occurred. The psychological effects of chemotherapy may vary according to the stage of disease at which it is prescribed.

Had the control group in the present study not received radiotherapy, would excess psychological morbidity due to chemotherapy have emerged before 13 months? Radiotherapy has been thought perhaps to increase psychological morbidity following mastectomy, either because it implies a worse prognosis or because of its de-energizing effect (Maguire et al., 1978; Greer, 1985). However, in a controlled study comparing post-operative radiotherapy with no further treatment in 85 mastectomy patients, the authors and colleagues found radiotherapy to be associated with significant excesses of somatic symptoms and social dysfunction, but not with any appreciable excess of depression or anxiety (Hughson et al., 1987). Although certain patients found that radiotherapy provoked anxiety, others became anxious through not receiving any further treatment. The study of Cassileth et al. (1986), referred to above, also suggests that not having further therapy may induce anxiety. Receiving post-operative treatment may sometimes in itself be reassuring, and usually results in patients being seen frequently by professional staff. Any adverse psychological effects of treatment may thus be counteracted, unless the treatment is especially long or arduous.

Finally, the present study provides no information on the effects on patients' relatives of the decision to prescribe adjuvant chemotherapy. This apparently simple question presents an immense challenge for future research.

ACKNOWLEDGEMENTS

Results of this study, supported by the Cancer Research Campaign, were originally published in the British Medical Journal.* We are grateful to the publishers of the British Medical Journal for permission to reproduce material. We thank the patients for their prolonged co-operation, and the following people for permission to interview those under their care: members of the Division of Surgery, Victoria

*See References.

Infirmary, Glasgow; Professor K. C. Calman of the Department of Clinical Oncology, Gartnavel General Hospital, Glasgow, Drs Agnes Russell and Tim Habeshaw of the Institute of Radiotherapeutics and Oncology, Western Infirmary, Glasgow. We also thank Dr Peter Maguire, Senior Lecturer in Psychiatry, University of Manchester, who kindly allowed us to use his rating scales, and our surgical colleagues, Mr Colin McArdle and Mr David Smith.

REFERENCES

Anonymous (1984) Review of mortality results in randomised trials in early breast cancer [Editorial]. *Lancet* **ii**, 1205.

Baum, M., Priestman, T., West, R. R. and Jones, E. M. (1980) A comparison of subjective responses in a trial comparing endocrine with cytotoxic treatment in advanced carcinoma of the breast. *Eur. J. Cancer* **Suppl. 1** 223–226.

Bonadonna, G., Brusamolino, E., Valagussa, P., Rossi, A., Brugnatelli, L., Brambilla, C., De Lena, M., Tancini, G., Bajetta, E., Musumeci, R. and Veronesi, U. (1976) Combination chemotherapy as an adjuvant treatment in operable breast cancer. *New Engl. J. Med.* **294**, 405–410.

Bonadonna, G., Valagussa, P., Rossi, A., Tancini, G., Brambilla, C., Zambetti, M. and Veronesi, U. (1985) Ten-year experience with CMF-based adjuvant chemotherapy in resectable breast cancer. *Breast Cancer Res. Treat.* **5**, 95–115.

Cassileth, B. R., Knuiman, M. W., Abeloff, M. D., Falkson, G., Ezdinli, E. Z. and Mehta, C. R. (1986). Anxiety levels in patients randomized to adjuvant therapy versus observation for early breast cancer. *J. Clin. Onco.* **4**, 972–974.

Cohen, J. (1968) Weighted kappa: nominal scale agreement with provision for scaled disagreement or partial credit. *Psychol. Bull.* **70**, 213–220.

Consensus Conference (1985) Adjuvant chemotherapy for breast cancer. *J. Am. Med. Assoc.* **254**, 3461–3463.

Goldberg, D. P., (1979) *Manual of the General Health Questionnaire*. NFER, Windsor.

Greer, S. (1985) Cancer, psychiatric aspects. In, Granville-Grossman, K., ed. *Recent Advances in Clinical Psychiatry*, pp. 87–104. Churchill Livingstone, Edinburgh.

Howell, A., George, W. D., Crowther, D., Rubens, R. D., Bulbrook, R. D., Bush, H., Howat, J. M. T., Sellwood, R., Hayward, J. L., Fentiman, I. S. and Chaudary, M. (1984) Controlled trial of adjuvant chemotherapy with cyclophosphamide, methotrexate, and fluorouracil for breast cancer. *Lancet* **ii**, 307–311.

Hughson, A. V. M., Cooper, A. F., McArdle, C. S., Russell, A. R. and Smith, D. C. (1980) Psychiatric morbidity in disease-free survivors following radiotherapy and adjuvant chemotherapy for breast cancer: a 2-year follow-up study. *Br. J. Surg.* **67**, 370.

Hughson, A. V. M., Cooper, A. F., McArdle, C. S. and Smith, D. C. (1986) Psychological impact of adjuvant chemotherapy in the first two years after mastectomy. *Br. Med. J.* **293**, 1268–1271.

Hughson, A. V. M., Cooper, A. F., McArdle, C. S. and Smith D. C. (1987) Psychosocial effects of radiotherapy after mastectomy. *Br. Med. J.*, **294**, 1515–1518.

Knobf, M. K. (1986) Physical and psychologic distress associated with adjuvant chemotherapy in women with breast cancer. *J. Clin. Oncol.* **4**, 678–684.

McArdle, C. S., Crawford, D., Dykes, E. E., Calman, K. C., Hole, D., Russell, A. R. and Smith, D. C. (1986) Adjuvant radiotherapy and chemotherapy in breast cancer. *Br. J. Surg.* **73**, 264–266.

Maguire, G. P., Lee, E. G., Bevington, D. J., Küchemann, C., Crabtree, R. J. and Cornell, C. (1978) Psychiatric problems in the first year after mastectomy. *Br. Med. J.* **i**, 963–965

Maguire, G. P., Tait, A., Brooke, M., Thomas, C., Howat, J. M. T. and Sellwood, R. (1980) Psychiatric morbidity and physical toxicity associated with adjuvant chemotherapy after mastectomy. *Br. Med. J.* **281**, 1179–1180.

Meyerowitz, B. E., Sparks, F. C., Spears, I. K. (1979) Adjuvant chemotherapy for breast carcinoma: Psychosocial implications. *Cancer* **43**, 1613–1618.

Meyerowitz, B. E., Watkins, I. K. and Sparks, F. C. (1983) Psychosocial implications of adjuvant chemotherapy. A two-year follow-up. *Cancer* **52**, 1541–1545.

Neese, R., Corli, T., Curtis, G. and Kleinman, P. (1980) Pretreatment nausea in cancer chemotherapy: a conditioned response? *Psychosom. Med.* **58**, 277–299.

Palmer, B. V., Walsh, G. A., McKinna, J. A. and Greening, W. P. (1980) Adjuvant chemotherapy for breast cancer: side-effects and quality of life. *Br. Med. J.* **281**, 1594–1597.

Silberfarb, P. M., Maurer, L. H., Crouthamel, C. (1980) Psychosocial aspects of neoplastic disease: I. Functional status of breast cancer patients during different treatment regimens. *Am. J. Psychia.* **137**, 450–455.

Snaith, R. P., Bridge, G. W. and Hamilton, M. (1976) The Leeds scales for the self assessment of anxiety and depression. *Br. J. Psychia.* **128**, 156–165.

Velpeau, A., trans. by Henry, M. (1856). *A Treatise on the Diseases of the Breast and Mammary Region.* Sydenham Society, London.

Psychological Effects of the Offer of Breast Reconstruction following Mastectomy

R. GLYNN OWENS, J. J. ASHCROFT, P. D. SLADE AND S. J. LEINSTER

ABSTRACT

Twenty-five women, for whom mastectomy was considered a necessary treatment for their cancer, were offered breast reconstruction to be completed on the same day as the breast removal. Eight women accepted this offer, and these patients tended to be younger and more concerned about appearance and the disease than those who refused it. All patients appreciated being given some control over their treatment and said in interview that this helped them cope. Tests of depression, anxiety, body satisfaction, marital adjustment, self-esteem, sociability and life change were given prior to surgery and at intervals up to 1 year after. Psychosocial adaption was good in all patients. It is suggested that the offer of breast reconstruction, wherever technically feasible, is a positive step towards ensuring psychological well-being of mastectomy patients.

A large number of studies have indicated psychological distress consequent upon mastectomy (Meyerowitz, 1980). Inevitably, precise estimates of incidence are to some extent a function of the criteria used by investigators and the methodological rigour of individual studies. Nevertheless a comparison of independent studies (Maguire, 1985) has noted broad agreement amongst researchers, with reports of around 20% for the incidence of anxiety and depression. Moreover Maguire *et al.* (1978) noted that mastectomy patients were almost four times as likely as patients with benign disease to report a marked lessening in sexual desire and enjoyment, with serious problems apparent in a third of the mastectomy patients. Whilst such problems as depression may be similarly common in patients with other types of cancer (Worden & Weisman, 1977) a considerable amount of circumstantial and clinical evidence suggests that mastectomy itself may contribute to the patients' psychological problems. Morris *et al.* (1977) note difficulty in adapting to disfigurement in a large percentage of mastectomy patients even one year after surgery, with similar results being reported by Maguire *et al.* (1983). Attempts to identify which individuals are at risk of developing subsequent problems have, perhaps unsurprisingly, indicated concern about disfigurement or ugliness as predictors (Ray, 1977; Metzger *et al.*, 1983).

A logical step in the light of such studies is to attempt to lessen the effect of breast loss by the provision of surgical breast reconstruction. Chaglassian and Sherman (1983) review a number of techniques by which a reconstructed breast can be provided, remarking that such techniques are becoming increasingly refined, satisfactory and acceptable to both the public and the medical community. A controlled trial of reconstruction using a prosthetic implant has suggested that such a procedure may reduce anxiety and depression (Dean *et al.*, 1983). Practitioners involved in reconstruction procedures have commonly remarked on the need for careful selection of women offered such an option (England, 1985; Chaglassian & Sherman, 1983). The basis for such selection however has yet to be systematically investigated. In the absence of any basis for such selection it may be seen as appropriate to offer reconstruction to all mastectomy patients. A recent study at the Royal Liverpool Hospital showed improved psychological outcome in patients offered a choice of treatment, mastectomy or lumpectomy plus radiotherapy (Ashcroft *et al.*, 1985). Of relevance to the present issue is that even where appearance was of relatively little importance and patients chose mastectomy, the fact that women were responsible for their choice appeared to help them to cope. As a consequence of such findings it was postulated that where choice of treatment could not be offered, (mastectomy being necessary on medical grounds) the psychological morbidity might be lessened if women were once again given the opportunity to choose for themselves. The present paper reports our initial findings regarding the effect of offering such a choice.

METHOD

Subjects

Subjects were 25 mastectomy patients from a wide range of social class undergoing treatment at the Royal Liverpool Hospital; mean age was 55 years (S.D. 11 years).

Instruments

The following assessments were used:
(i)   The Leeds Scales (Snaith *et al.*, 1977), for the measurement of anxiety and depression.
(ii)   The Spielberger State-Trait Anxiety Inventory (Spielberger *et al.*, 1970).
(iii)   Body Satisfaction Scales.
(iv)   Social Adaptability (Watson and Friend 1969).
(v)   The Marital Adjustment Test (Locke and Wallace 1959).
(vi)   Self Esteem (Dohrenwend *et al.*, 1980).

(vii)   Life Events (Holmes and Rahe, 1967).
(viii)   Ratings of degree of concern (1-10 scale) about appearance, disease and treatment.

Procedure

The offer was made of breast reconstruction using a procedure whereby the chest wall is reconstructed from back muscle (latissimus dorsi musculocutaneous flap) to form the new breast mound, with the addition of a prosthesis as necessary. The surgeon explained the procedure and its likely physical effects. The possibility of additional surgery at a later date for recreation of the nipple–areola complex was also discussed. Where the woman opted for reconstruction this was carried out at the same time as the mastectomy.

The psychological assessments listed above were all given the day before surgery and at 3 month and 1 year follow-up. Three days after surgery additional questionnaires relating to depression and anxiety were given. In addition a questionnaire was sent at both follow-up periods which asked direct questions about level of activity, personal relationships and health (including degree of satisfaction with reconstruction where this was applicable). Patients were also interviewed the day before surgery, at which time they were asked to give the ratings of degree of concern regarding appearance, disease and treatment; patients were also interviewed before they left hospital.

RESULTS

Acceptance of the offer

Of the 25 women offered breast reconstruction, eight (32%) took up this option.

Age

Women accepting the offer of reconstruction were significantly (f = 32.99, P<0.001) younger (mean age 43 years, S.D. 8 years) than those declining (mean age 61 years, S.D. 7 years).

Ratings of concern

Women accepting the offer of reconstruction were significantly (f = 15.4, P<0.001) more concerned about appearance (mean rating 8, S.D. 2.3) than those who declined (mean rating 3.6, S.D. 2.7). Those accepting were also significantly (f = 5.26, P<0.05) more concerned about the disease (mean rating 8.8, S.D. 1.8) than those who declined (mean rating 6.1, S.D. 3.1).

Other measures

No other sustained difference was found between the groups on any of the measures taken either during the interview or via formal testing. Three days post operatively those choosing reconstruction showed significantly (f = 4.54, $P < 0.05$) more anxiety on the Spielberger State Trait Anxiety Inventory (mean score 46.1, S.D. 7.0) than those who declined (mean score 37.4, S.D. 9.7). This difference did not however persist and was not apparent at follow-up. Generally, scores for both groups showed then to be slightly anxious and depressed when knowledge of cancer was first discussed. However, adaptation to treatment was generally excellent, without the profound psychosocial problems previously reported in the literature.

DISCUSSION

Interpretation of results such as these is generally considered problematic by comparison with the results of randomized trials. In an area like breast reconstruction however it should be remembered that randomization is itself not without its difficulties. Perhaps foremost amongst these is the ethical issue of witholding of treatment; if the present study had been conducted on a randomization basis, approximately half of the women participating would have been denied reconstruction. The problem is not necessarily solved by the principle of "informed consent". Whilst giving women the choice of whether or not to participate in randomization has an intuitive appeal, the results of such a procedure in practice may be far from satisfactory. It has been the practice at Liverpool to ensure that women offered the opportunity to participate in "a random trial" fully appreciate what is meant by randomization, explaining that in effect this means that a decision will be made as if by the toss of a coin. Our experience has been that few women to whom a full explanation is given wish to give over such an important decision to a random process. A consequence of this is that the use of an ethically justifiable procedure brings its own methodological difficulties in that the few who do decide to participate are unlikely to be representative of all patients. In the randomized trial reported by Dean et al. (1983) for example, it is notable that almost half of the women approached refused to take part in the trial. It can be argued therefore that there is a place for the non-randomized trial in which the representativeness of the sample compensates for the difficulties in comparison.

An additional problem with randomization is evident in considering eventual comparisons. Whilst it is commonly assumed that the no-treatment group constitutes a "control", it must be remembered that their experience of the trial is not that of a normal patient. In particular, if a women wakes up after the operation to find that she was one of the "unlucky" ones denied reconstruction, this may itself have unfortunate psychological consequences. Such an effect may artificially inflate the benefits perceived in the experimental group.

In the present study it is clear from the results that the women who chose reconstruction were younger, more concerned about their appearance, and more concerned about the presence of cancer. Whilst the first two findings may appear fairly obvious, the relevance of concern with cancer is less so. One possible interpretation is that part of women's overall concern with cancer was itself related to concerns about appearance. That is to say, cancer is a cause of worry not only because of its life-threatening nature but additionally because of the threat to appearance. Such an interpretation can at this time, however, remain only speculative. It is notable, moreover, that despite the more extensive surgery involved in reconstruction, concerns about treatment were not elevated in this group. All those who chose reconstruction reported relief that something could be done to help them preserve their appearance, and all except one rated satisfaction with their reconstruction highly (8 or above on a 1–10 scale) at follow-up. The one woman who was not satisfied was offered, and accepted, further surgery to improve her appearance.

Perhaps the most striking feature of the results reported here is the general satisfaction expressed by all the women, irrespective of whether or not they chose reconstruction. Such satisfaction was expressed even where the degree of post-operative discomfort was marked. Whilst many factors may be adduced to account for such positive results, the opportunity for women to exercise some degree of control over their treatment may be of particular significance. All patients voiced their thanks of the offer of reconstruction, even when this option was not taken up, and it would certainly seem that having a degree of control helped the women to adapt well. The notion that control may affect both anxiety (e.g. Estes and Skinner, 1941) and depression (e.g. Seligman, 1975) has of course received considerable support in experimental psychology. In addition the results are of course consistent with those reported earlier regarding the role of patient choice in treatment (Ashcroft *et al.*, 1985). The results therefore further support the notion that giving patients increased control over their treatment may be associated with improved psychological outcome.

REFERENCES

Ashcroft, J. J., Leinster, S. and Slade, P. D. (1985) Breast cancer – patient choice of treatment: preliminary communication. *J. Roy. Soc. Med.* **78**, 43–46.

Chaglassian, T. A. and Sherman, J. E. (1983) Breast reconstruction after mastectomy. Margoles, R. G., ed Breast Cancer: Contemporary Issues in Clinical Oncology, Vol. 1, Churchhill Livingstone, London.

Dean, C., Chetty, U. and Forrest, A. P. M. (1983) Effects of immediate breast reconstruction on psychosocial morbidity after mastectomy. Lancet i, 459–462.

Dohrenwend, B. P., Shrout, P. E., Egri, G. and Mendelsohn, F. S. (1980) Non specific psychological distress and other dimensions of psychopathology. Arch. Gen. Psychiat. 37, 1229–1236.

England, P. C. (1985) Reconstruction of the breast. Tobias, J. S. and Peckham M. J., ed, Primary Management of Breast Cancer; Alternatives to Mastectomy, Edward Arnold, London, 1985.

Estes, W. K. and Skinner, B. F. (1941) Some quantitative properties of anxiety. J. Exp. Psycholo. 29, 390–400.

Holmes, T. H. and Rahe, R. H. (1967) The social readjustment rating scale. J. Psychosoma. Res. 11, 213–218.

Locke, H. J. and Wallace, K. M. (1959) Short term marital adjustment and prediction tests; their reliability and validity. Marriage Fam. Living 251.

Maguire, P. (1985) Psychological aspects of mastectomy. In Tobias, J. S. and Peckham, M. J. eds Primary Management of Breast Cancer; Alternatives to Mastectomy, Edward Arnold, London.

Maguire, G. P., Lee, E. G., Bevington, D. J., Kickemann, C. S., Crabtree,. R. J. and Cornell, C. E. (1978) Psychiatric problems in the first year after mastectomy. Br. Med. J. 1, 963–965.

Maguire, P. Brooke, M., Tait, A., Thomas, C. and Sellwood, R. (1983) Effect of counselling on the physical disability and social recovery after mastectomy. Clin. Oncol. 9, 319–324.

Metzger, L. F., Rogers, T. F. and Bauman, L. J. (1983) Effects of age and marital status on emotional distress after mastectomy. J. Psychosoc. Oncol. 1, 17.

Meyerowitz, B. E. (1980) Psychosocial correlates of breast cancer and its treatment, Psycholo. Bull. 87, 108–131.

Morris, T., Greer, H. S. and White, P. (1977) Psychological and social adjustment to mastectomy; a two-year follow-up study. Cancer 40, 2381–2387.

Ray, C. (1977) Psychological implications of mastectomy. Br. J. Soc. Clin. Psychol. 16, 373–377.

Seligman, M. E. P. (1975) Helplessness; on Depression, Development and Death, W. H. Freeman, San Francisco.

Snaith, R. P., Bridge, G. W. K. and Hamilton, M. (1977) The Leeds Scale for self-assessment of anxiety and depression. Psychological Test Publications, Barnstaple.

Spielberger C. D., Gorsuch, R. L. and Lushene, K. E. (1970) State–trait Anxiety Inventory Manual, Consulting Psychologist Press, Palo Alto, California.

Watson, D. and Friend, R. (1969) Measurement of social evaluative anxiety. J. Consult. Clin. Psychol. 33, 448–457.

Worden, W. J. and Weisman, A. D. (1977) The fallacy in post mastectomy depression. Am. J. Med. Sci. 73, 169–175.

Psychological Consequences of the Diagnosis and Management of Cancer: A Physician's View

CHRISTOPHER J. WILLIAMS

Although clinicians have tried to assess the impact of their treatment on cancer in prospective randomized controlled trials, it is very much more difficult to quantify the psychosocial consequences of the disease and its management. Despite the use of controlled clinical trials for the development of new anticancer therapies, only general rules about treatment can be formulated. For instance, a trial may show (Fig. 1) that treatment A is more effective than B in two randomly chosen groups, each of 100 patients. What such a study does not necessarily tell you, is which treatment is best for the next patient you see with this condition. The best that can be said is that treatment A gives the best overall chance of long term survival. Since studies of the psychosocial impact of cancer and its treatment are perhaps more difficult to formulate and run than trials of anticancer treatment and because variation from one patient and their family to another may be great, it can be seen that it is difficult to design a strategy for helping an individual cancer patient.

However, one approach may be to try to devise practical ways of identifying those at risk of developing major problems so that attempts to help can be targeted at those likely to be in most need. A further important area is to identify and reduce as far as possible some of the causes of stress. This chapter will briefly review some of the data regarding these two approaches, concentrating on breast cancer because the great majority of work has been in this area.

Identifying those at risk

There is little doubt that most if not all patients with cancer suffer a variety of psychosocial problems, though many reports have concentrated on particular aspects of diagnosis or treatment. Maguire and his colleagues (Maguire, 1976; Maguire et al., 1978) and others (Hughes, 1982; Beckmann et al., 1983) have reported on the psychiatric morbidity associated with breast cancer surgery, principally

119

Christopher J. Williams

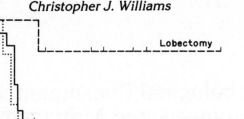

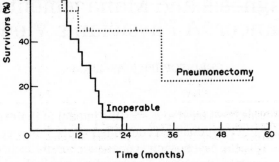

Time (months)

FIG. 1. ACTUARIAL SURVIVAL ACCORDING TO SURGICAL
PROCEDURE AFTER THREE INITIAL CYCLES OF
COMBINATION CHEMOTHERAPY. ALTHOUGH PATIENTS
UNDERGOING A LOBECTOMY FARED SIGNIFICANTLY BETTER
THAN THOSE HAVING A PNEUMONECTOMY OR INOPERABLE
PATIENTS, SUCH A RESULT DOES NOT ALLOW YOU TO
DECIDE WHETHER SURGERY IS THE BEST TREATMENT FOR
THE NEWLY DIAGNOSED CASE OF THE DISEASE.

mastectomy (Table 1). In Maguire's original study the control group consisted of women with benign breast disease, and it is, therefore, not surprising that anxiety, depression and sexual problems were more common (34%) in the breast cancer group. However, in the study of Worden and Weisman (1977) there was no evidence of post-mastectomy depression in 40 women; the control group in this study being 30 women with other types of cancer. Clearly, though mastectomy *per se* may have caused some mood disturbances, a large element of the anxiety and depression was directly related to the finding of cancer and all that that entailed in the patient's mind.

Although a majority of patients in the studies of Maguire *et al.* (1976, 1978) had some measurable degree of anxiety and depression, only about one-third had moderate to severe problems. His next study (Maguire *et al.*, 1980) was, therefore, designed to see if these patients could be identified early in an attempt to reduce the impact of the patient's problems. In this well known randomized study, he chose to use specialist nurses as counsellors to a group of patients chosen at random and compared the psychosocial problems in this group with those in patients managed routinely in the same clinic. Depression, anxiety and sexual problems were independently assessed by a psychiatrist at 3 months and 12–18 months after surgery. Seventy five patients were counselled by

TABLE 1. MOOD CHANGES IN FIRST YEAR AFTER MASTECTOMY (MAGUIRE ET AL. 1978)

Severity of mood change	Four months		Twelve months	
	No. mastectomy group (%)	No. control (%)	No. mastectomy group (%)	No. control (%)
Anxiety*				
None	32 (43)	32 (68)	28 (37)	32 (64)
Minor	27 (36)	12 (24)	33 (44)	14 (28)
Moderate	14 (18)	4 (8)	12 (16)	4 (8)
Severe	2 (3)	— —	2 (3)	— —
Depression†				
None	31 (41)	32 (64)	31 (41)	35 (70)
Minor	24 (32)	12 (24)	28 (38)	11 (22)
Moderate	19 (26)	6 (12)	11 (15)	4 (8)
Severe	1 (1)	— —	5 (7)	— —

*anxiety: comparison between mastectomy and control groups for none vs. some symptoms, at 4 months $P < 0.01$ and at 1 year $P < 0.01$.
†depression: comparison between mastectomy and control groups for none vs. some symptoms, at 4 months $P < 0.05$ and at 1 year $P < 0.01$.

the nurse and 77 had routine care only. Counselling failed to prevent morbidity at 3 months after mastectomy, but the nurse was able to recognize problems in 34 of 38 women (89%) compared with only 9 of 41 (22%) recognized by those concerned in routine care. Following recognition of problems, 29 of the 34 women in the counselled group were referred for additional psychiatric care. The apparent result of this was to reduce the levels of problems in the counselled group when these were measured 12–18 months postoperatively (Table 2). Whilst nurse counselling reduced psychiatric problems and speeded social recovery it had no effect on physical disability (Maguire *et al.*, 1983). The incidence of significant psychosocial morbidity in this study was particularly high (39%); a finding related by the authors to the large number of patients receiving adjuvant chemotherapy.

Several studies have strongly suggested that adjuvant chemotherapy significantly increases the risk of psychiatric morbidity after initial breast cancer surgery (Cooper *et al.*, 1979; Meyerowitz *et al.*, 1979, 1983; Maguire *et al.*, 1980; Nerenz *et al.*, 1982; Palmer *et al.*, 1980). Since current patterns of management have become increasingly complicated, patients receiving prolonged therapy are likely to be at high risk of developing psychiatric problems. For instance a pre-menopausal woman with T_{1-2}, N_1, M_0 breast tumour may well be treated with a lumpectomy followed by a fairly prolonged course of radiation to the breast and then six cycles of CMF adjuvant chemotherapy.

The need for adjuvant therapy may be associated with distress since it underlines that the patient has an increased risk of tumour recurrence. On top of this, the physical side effects of chemotherapy are sufficient to cause psychosocial morbidity themselves (Nerenz *et al.*, 1982). The use of such adjuvant therapy should therefore alert the clinician and

TABLE 2. PSYCHIATRIC MORBIDITY AT 3 AND 12-18 MONTHS AFTER MASTECTOMY: EFFECT OF COUNSELLING BY A SPECIALIST NURSE. MAGUIRE ET AL. 1980

Degree of morbidity	% Anxiety State*		% Depression†		% Sexual Problems‡	
	Counselled	Routine	Counselled	Routine	Counselled	Routine
Morbidity 3 months after mastectomy						
Absent	69	68	68	69	60	69
Mild	15	16	11	14	—	—
Moderately severe	11	10	18	16	10	12
Severe	5	6	3	1	30	19
Morbidity 12-18 months after mastectomy						
Absent	92	70	95	70	92	69
Mild	5	8	1	10	—	—
Moderately severe	3	19	4	17	6	23
Severe	0	3	0	3	2	8

*comparison counselled and routine $P < 0.01$
†comparison counselled and routine $P < 0.001$
‡comparison counselled and routine $P < 0.02$

mastectomy nurse to the potential risk of distress in these patients. Such information also suggests that every effort should be made to prevent or reduce the subjective toxicities of chemotherapy. Among the most distressing is nausea and vomiting (Williams, 1984) and Nerenz et al. (1982) found a particularly high level of distress in patients who developed conditioned vomiting. In addition to ensuring the best antiemetic cover from the outset it is important that the environment and staff dealing with the patient are perceived as "friendly". The administration of chemotherapy by one approachable individual (preferably a chemotherapy nurse) in comfortable surroundings will do much to allay anxiety and reduces the tension that becomes associated with the "ritual" of giving chemotherapy. This may help to lessen anxiety and prevent conditioning.

Thus, studies of cancer patients have identified a significant proportion of patients who are severely distressed; patients at greater risk can be selected out and early identification and support may reduce the duration of distress that almost inevitably accompanies diagnosis and initial treatment.

REDUCING THE CAUSES OF STRESS

Delay in making the diagnosis

Studies have suggested that the period between recognizing an abnormality that may be cancer and being told the diagnosis is, not surprisingly, very stressful (Jamison et al., 1978). Of those discovering a breast lump in this study, the mean interval to examination by a doctor was 23 days (median 6 days). The mean interval being skewed by about 10% of women who delayed consultation. However, the mean interval between first medical consultation and biopsy, 27 days (median 10 days), was surprisingly long and exceeded delay by the patient. Every effort should be made to ensure that the period between first visit to a doctor and making a definitive diagnosis is as short as possible. Patients who imagine they may have cancer clearly need to be handled with great sensitivity and investigations and procedures planned as *quickly* and *simply* as possible.

Uncertainty over the diagnosis and treatment

Traditional patterns of breast cancer management have included frozen section biopsy which proceed to mastectomy if cancer is confirmed, or open biopsy followed at a later date by second stage surgery. More recently, the use of physical examination, mammography, ultrasound, and fine needle aspiration cytology often allows a definitive diagnosis to be made without a formal surgical procedure (Smallwood *et al.*, 1984). As a result of this policy, a diagnosis of breast cancer was made in over 80% of patients within 1 – 2 days from their first visit to a clinic. Patients with cancer and their families then have time to discuss the type of surgery that may be appropriate for them.

Discussing the treatment options

There is conflicting evidence about whether the use of lumpectomy reduces the levels of distress in the first post-operative year (Beckmann *et al.*, 1983; Schain *et al.*, 1983; Steinberg *et al.*, 1985; Ashcroft *et al.*, 1985; Bartelink *et al.*, 1985). Part of the problem for such studies has been finding a suitable control group; even in randomized series patients may not be truly representative, since they must be willing to accept either lumpectomy or mastectomy.

Some surgeons have viewed open discussion about the uncertainties regarding types of surgery available as threatening: considering that patients may think of them as indecisive if they do not recommend one therapy as best. There have also been doubts as to whether patients will worry if a definitive treatment plan is not presented to them. However, recent research in Southampton (Morris, 1987) has suggested that open discussion of the surgical options may well reduce anxiety and depression in the breast cancer patient and her spouse. In this preliminary study, the proportions of patients with moderately severe depression and anxiety (> 11 on the HAD scale) were recorded before surgery and 2 to 3 months later in four groups of patients. Group 1 had small resectable tumours beneath the nipple which were not suitable for mastectomy: these patients were told that they must have a mastectomy. Group 2 consisted of women who were suitable for lumpectomy: the

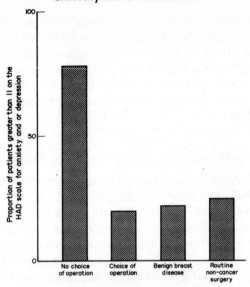

FIG. 2. PROPORTION OF PATIENTS SCORING
GREATER THAN 11 ON THE HAD SCALE FOR
ANXIETY AND/OR DEPRESSION. PATIENTS ARE
DIVIDED INTO FOUR SURGICAL GROUPS CONSISTING
OF, A) THOSE GIVEN NO CHOICE OF OPERATION
(MASTECTOMY BECAUSE OF SUBAREOLAR SITE OF
TUMOUR), B) PATIENTS GIVEN A CHOICE BETWEEN
WIDE EXCISION AND RADIOTHERAPY OR
MASTECTOMY, C) BIOPSY FOR BENIGN BREAST
DISEASE, D) ROUTINE NON-CANCER SURGERY.

situation was discussed openly and the patient allowed to decide on the type of surgery (lumpectomy or mastectomy) with medical advice, or following discussion they asked the surgeon to decide for them. Group 3 consisted of patients with benign breast disease and group 4 patients undergoing routine non-cancer surgery. The preliminary results (shown graphically in Fig. 2) strongly suggest that both anxiety and depression were significantly less of a problem in cancer patients who partook in discussions regarding their treatment (group 2), when compared with those who were told they must have a mastectomy (group 1). Although this is a small preliminary study, it shows that patients allowed to participate in the choice of their therapy were *not* compromised by this. If these data can be extrapolated to other situations, they suggest that patients do want to be a partner in making treatment decisions: a fact often reiterated by patients in clinic.

Attempts to lessen the psychosocial impact of the diagnosis and management of cancer are in their infancy. Up till now, studies have been phenomenological in character and only general advice can be given. Much of this is of a commonsense nature and includes:

(i)   Make the diagnosis as quickly as possible using simple non-invasive tests where possible.

(ii)   Explain the situation as fully as possible to patients and allow them to partake in making decisions: do not force decisions on them if they do not want this.

(iii) Give treatment in a "friendly atmosphere" where the patient has a chance to get to know and trust the staff. Use mastectomy nurses and chemotherapy nurses where possible: they are often able to form a closer relationship with patients.

(iv)   Make every attempt to reduce treatment related side effects.

(v)   Expect that a third or more of patients will have at least moderately severe mood change and sexual problems. The incidence of psychosocial problems is likely to be greater when complex and prolonged treatments are used.

(vi)   Early intervention and, when appropriate, psychiatric referral may lessen the period of severe morbidity.

REFERENCES

Ashcroft, J. J. Leinster, S. J. and Slade, P. D. (1985) Breast cancer – patient choice of treatment: preliminary communication. *J. Roy. Soc. Med.* **78**, 43–46.

Bartelink, H., van Dam, F., and van Dongen, J. (1985) Psychological effects of breast conserving therapy in comparison with radical mastectomy. *Int, J. Radiat. Oncol. Biol. Physi.* **11**, 381–385.

Beckmann, J., Johansen, L., Richardt, C., and Blichert-Toft, M. (1983) Psychological reactions in younger women operated on for breast cancer. *Dan. Med. Bull.* **30**, 10–13.

Cooper, A. F., McArdle, C. S., Russell, A. R., and Smith, D. C. (1979) Psychotic morbidity associated with adjuvant chemotherapy following mastectomy for breast cancer. *Brit. J. Surg.* **66**, 362 (abstr).

Hughes, J. (1982) Emotional reactions to the diagnosis and treatment of early breast cancer. *J. Psychosoma. Res.* **26**, 277–283.

Jamison, K. R., Wellisch, D. K., and Pasnan, R. O. (1978) Psychosocial aspects of mastectomy: 1, The woman's perspective. *Am. J. Psychia.* **135**, 432–436.

Maguire, G. P. (1976) The psychiatric and social sequelae of mastectomy. In Howles, J. G., ed., *Modern perspectives in the psychiatric aspects of surgery.* pp. 390–420, Brunner Mazel, New York.

Maguire, G. P., Brooke, M., Tait, A., Thomas, C., and Sellwood, R. (1983) The effect of counselling on physical disability and social recovery after mastectomy. *Clin. Oncol.* **9**, 319–324.

Maguire, G. P., Lee, E. G., Bevington, D. J., Kuchemann, C. S., Crabtree, R. J., and Cornell, C. E. (1978) Psychiatric problems in the first year after mastectomy. *Br. Med. J.* **i**, 963–965.

Maguire, G. P., Tait, A., Brooke, M., Thomas, C., Howat, J. M. T., Sellwood, R. A., and Bush, H. (1980) Psychiatric morbidity and physical toxicity associated with adjuvant chemotherapy after mastectomy. *Br. Med. J.* **281**, 1179–1180.

Maguire, P., Tait, A., Brooke, M., Thomas, C., Sellwood, R. (1980) Effect of counselling on the psychiatric morbidity associated with mastectomy. *Br. Med. J.* **281**, 1454–1456.

Meyerowitz, B. E., Sparks, F. C., Spears, I. K. (1979) Adjuvant chemotherapy for breast cancer: psychosocial implications. *Cancer* **43**, 1613–1618.

Meyerowitz, B. E. Watkins, I. K., Sparks, F. C. (1983) Quality of life for breast cancer patients receiving adjuvant chemotherapy. *Am. J. Nurs.* 232–235.

Morris, J. (1987) Personal communication.

Nerenz, D. R., Leventhal, H., and Love, R. R. (1982) Factors contributing to emotional distress during cancer chemotherapy. *Cancer* **50**, 1020–1027.

Palmer, B. V., Walsh, G. A., McKinna, J. A., and Greening, W. P. (1980) Adjuvant chemotherapy for breast cancer: side effects and quality of life. *Br. Med. J.* **281**, 1594–1597.

Schain, W., Edwards, B. K., and Rice Govvell, C. (1983) Psychosocial and physical outcomes of primary breast cancer therapy: mastectomy vs. excisional biopsy and irradiation. *Breast Cancer Res. Treat.* **3**, 377–382.

Smallwood, J., Khong, Y., and Boyd, A. (1984) Assessment of a scoring system for the preoperative diagnosis of breast lumps. *Ann. Roy. Coll. Surg. Eng.* **66**, 267–269.

Steinberg, M. D., Juliano, M. A., and Wise, L. (1985) Psychosocial outcome of lumpectomy versus mastectomy in the treatment of breast cancer *Am. J. Psychiat.* **142**, 34–39.

Williams, C. J. (1984) The management of nausea and vomiting by anticancer chemotherapy. In Harrup, K., ed., *The Biological Characterisation of Cancer.* Martinus Nijhoff, Amsterdam.

Worden, J. W., and Weisman, A. D. (1977) The fallacy of post mastectomy depression. *Am. J. Med. Sci.* **273**, 169–175.

The Impact of an Abnormal Cervical Smear

TINA POSNER

ABSTRACT

In medical terms, screening well women for abnormal cervical cells appears to be a triumph of preventative medicine: a serious disease can be prevented. However, the success of treatment has been judged entirely by the elimination of the abnormal cells and the absence of physical complications. The impact of the medical process of investigation and treatment following a positive or abnormal smear on the patient have not been sufficiently taken into account.

One hundred and fifty three women referred for investigations of abnormal or positive cervical smears were interviewed two or three times during the subsequent medical process. The first interview took place either just before or very soon after their first colposcopy examination; the last 6-9 months later, after any treatment needed had been carried out.

News of the abnormal smear result caused a considerable amount of alarm and anxiety. Most of the women at that stage thought of the cervical smear test in very black and white terms, so that if something was wrong, they assumed it was cancer. Few of the women had ever heard of colposcopy. More women mentioned this initial period prior to investigation as the most anxious period for them, than any other time. The colposcopy examination could provide a resolution of some, if not all, of the uncertainty and anxiety, and just over half (52%) of the patients felt better afterwards. However, 19% said they felt worse at the prospect of treatment, or because of continuing uncertainty or because of the stress of the examination. In the last interview, the women were asked how they would describe cancer. The majority of interviewees who felt able to describe cancer at all, talked in extremely negative, metaphorical terms of an unstoppable destruction of the human body and spirit. A third equated the disease with death or more figuratively "doom". Twenty-one percent talked of the body or more specifically, normal cells, being eaten away, devoured, invaded or destroyed by it. Only a minority of women described the disease in technical terms, mentioning cellular abnormalities or growth, or different types of cancer with different prognoses.

Though the women interviewed were knowledgeable about the curability of a specific cancer relevant to them, their picture of the disease in general remained dominated by the prevailing cultural image of the disease which presents it as essentially unbeatable. This image influenced their view of future health prospects and counterbalanced the knowledge they acquired (during the medical process of investigation and treatment), of the protective function of the cervical smear test and the essentially optimistic outlook with CIN. This meant that over half the sample were not confident that the threat of cancer represented by the abnormal cervical smear finding had altogether receded.

Several factors appeared to be particularly important in structuring women's perceptions after an abnormal cervical smear finding: lack of information, especially in the initial stages; the influence of a very negative and metaphorical image of cancer and stereotype of the sort of women likely to develop cervical cancer; and a feeling of being out of control of what was happening. It is recommended that more information be provided (in both verbal and written form) in order to: avoid unnecessary anxiety and stress; help prepare women for the colposcopy examination and any subsequent treatment and follow-up; fill the conceptual gap so that the image of cancer has less influence; and allow women to be more involved in discussions of the management of the health risk presented by the abnormal cervical cells so that they need not feel so out of control of what was happening to their bodies. Increased understanding of the nature of CIN and its treatment could help change the doom-laden image of cancer as a disease.

ACKNOWLEDGEMENTS

The research on which this paper is based was funded by the Cancer Research Campaign between 1982 and 1985, while the author was a research associate in the University of Oxford Department of Community Medicine and General Practice. The report of the study "Prevention of Cervical Cancer: The Patient's View", T. Posner and M. Vessey, is to be published by the King's Fund in 1988.

Use of a Simple Self-assessment Method to Measure Anxiety and Social Disturbance in Adults with Potentially Curable Malignant Disease

MARCIA A. RATCLIFFE, AUDREY A. DAWSON and
HOWARD WARING

ABSTRACT

Long-term disease-free survival after complete remission is the aim of the clinician in using aggressive chemotherapy in young adults with widespread or systemic lymphoma, or with teratoma. However, even in patients who achieve good remission or cure, the price in poor quality of life may be high.

The impact of being told that one has malignant disease is enormous, especially to a young patient. He is no longer shielded from the realities, since he will be told the diagnosis and proposed treatment. The clinician's concern is mainly with his physical well-being, regression of disease during his therapy and maintenance of complete remission afterwards. We aimed to identify those patients, long-term survivors of malignant disease, who were at most risk of an unnecessarily poor quality of life.

The method of measuring patient well being had to be simple, and capable of being carried out during clinic visits without upset even in the absence of psychological support. A simple linear analogue self assessment (LASA) method was adopted to measure (a) anxiety at the time of assessment, remembered anxiety at diagnosis and about treatment; (b) disturbance to life with respect to work, social and family life, sexual relations, and leisure pursuits, and (c) mood and life satisfaction. A total anxiety score and total social disturbance score were derived by amalgamating the scores in (a) and (b) respectively.

Of 84 adults between 18 and 50 years studied, all completed the LASA without upset, on average in 5 mins during waiting periods at the clinics, where patients on therapy and after therapy, were being examined and assessed.

Fifty-seven patients (26 males, 31 females) suffered from lymphoma, 17 were still on therapy, 40 had finished first-line day-patient therapy 6-60 months earlier; 27 had had a teratoma, all male, and nine were still having chemotherapy, 18 having finished therapy 6-60 months before.

Anxiety levels were high both in patients on and off treatment, and the time after treatment did not affect the levels.

No particular form of treatment, and no socio-demographic characteristics correlated with high anxiety levels, nor did dissatisfaction with medical information about the disease. However, the degree of self-assessed anxiety correlated well with one clinician's independent estimate of anxiety.

Social disturbance was highest in patients with teratoma having therapy, which was given intermittently as in-patient treatment, but, although social upset was still recorded in patients after stopping treatment, the groups of teratoma and

129

lymphoma patients off treatment nevertheless had a considerable reduction in disturbance.

In a small group of seven patients studied twice, these finding were confirmed.

Over half the patients expressed a wish to have had access to a support group, or to discussion with an ex-patient in the same clinical situation as himself. These facilities were not available at the time of the study, but are being set up now. Perhaps this will be one step towards allaying the anxiety (with accompanying low mood, and dissatisfaction with life) which has been shown by this simple LASA method to persist even though the patient has got back to a reasonable social pattern of life after successful treatment of cancer.

D. Psychological Intervention/Support

A Randomized Controlled Trial of Preoperative Psychological Preparation for Mastectomy. A Preliminary Report

MARY V. BURTON and RONALD W. PARKER

ABSTRACT

The effectiveness of a preoperative psychotherapeutic intervention with mastectomy patients is being assessed in an ongoing randomized controlled trial. Patients are assigned to one of four groups: (A) preoperative interview plus a 30-min preoperative psychotherapeutic intervention; (B) preoperative interview plus a 30-min chat to control for the effects of attention; (C) preoperative interview only; and (D) routine hospital care. A clinical psychologist administers the interview and a consultant surgeon trained in listening and counselling skills conducts a brief psychotherapeutic intervention based on data gathered from the interview. The intervention is designed to place the current crisis of the illness and surgery within the patient's life situation, and to provide an opportunity to explore feelings. The chat condition involves a friendly discussion of matters unrelated to the illness and surgery. Transcripts of chats and interventions are coded using Stiles' Verbal Response Modes in order to specify differences between them in modes of interpersonal interaction. Outcome is assessed by a Recovery Index on discharge and psychological functioning at 4 days, 3 months and 1 year postoperatively. Preliminary findings from the first 100 patients in the trial are presented. Patients receiving the preoperative psychotherapeutic intervention are experiencing less complicated recoveries than patients in control groups. Implications of the findings are discussed in the context of previous studies of psychological intervention with breast cancer patients.

There is now an extensive literature documenting the benefits of preoperative psychological preparation for surgery (Anderson and Masur, 1983; Cohen and Lazarus, 1973; Devine and Cook, 1983; Gil, 1984; Janis, 1983; Kendall, 1983; MacDonald and Kuiper, 1983; Mathews and Ridgeway, 1984; Mumford et al., 1982; Reading, 1979; Wilson, 1981). Evidence has accumulated that psychological preparation has a salutary effect not only on length of hospital stay but also on a wide range of physical recovery measures and postoperative psychological functioning. Methodological problems have been noted in most of the reviews, and our study has addressed many of these problems. There is a need for well-controlled studies, especially those designed to demonstrate the effectiveness of a brief psychotherapeutic interview. Most existing work has assessed the value of giving information about the procedures, information about the sensations the patient will experience during the procedure, relaxation training, or cognitive-behavioural interventions.

Mastectomy patients have been found to suffer a marked degree of postoperative psychological, social and sexual dysfunction (Asken, 1975; Beckmann et al., 1983; Gerard, 1982; Jamison et al., 1978, 1979; Maguire et al., 1978; Morris et al., 1977; Ray, 1977, 1978; Tait et al., 1982; Wellisch et al., 1978; Witkin, 1978). Several studies have described psychosocial interventions (Gordon et al., 1980; Maguire, 1984; Morganstern et al., 1984; Pfefferbaum et al., 1977–1978; Watson, 1983, Wellisch, 1984): the use of specialist nurses in assessing and counselling patients post-mastectomy (Faulkner and Maguire, 1984; Maguire et al., 1980a, 1983); self-help groups such as the Mastectomy Association (Kleiman et al., 1977; Tierney and Murrell, 1985; Wenderlin, 1978); cognitive behavioural therapy (Tarrier and Maguire, 1984; Tarrier et al., 1983); individual, marital and sexual therapy (Goldberg, 1981; Christenson, 1983; Vachon et al., 1981–1982; Witkin, 1975, 1978); and group therapy (Baider et al., 1984; Blake, 1984; Schwartz, 1977; Spiegel et al., 1981). In most of this work the focus has been on postoperative intervention.

Three recent studies of preoperative counselling with mastectomy patients have appeared in the nursing literature. Nurses have provided counselling which includes elements of information and emotional support (Baum and Jones, 1979; Lierman, 1982, 1984); or they have carried out an intervention roughly equivalent to our preoperative structured interview, without our preoperative psychotherapeutic intervention (Maguire et al., 1980b).

In another study (Gordon et al., 1980), preoperative interviews were followed by an individually tailored intervention for each patient, which included patient education and counselling. Or a combination of information, individual and group counselling was provided (Bloom et al., 1978). In our study, an attempt is made not only to encourage the expression of feelings and discuss coping efforts, but to discover the meaning of the current illness and surgery in the wider context of the patient's life situation and to explore this with the patient (Lazarus and Hagens, 1968; Streltzer and Leigh, 1978; Viederman and Perry, 1980; Worden and Weisman, 1984). Our intervention therefore goes beyond the more general "support" and "counselling" strategies reported in existing studies.

A wide variety of psychological variables have been studied in the surgical patient with a view to predicting those patients who will experience the most complicated recovery: locus of control, preoperative anxiety and depression, life stress, social support, and coping style are among them. Studies investigating the relationship between personality and surgical recovery have recently been reviewed (Cohen and Lazarus, 1973; Gil, 1984; Mathews and Ridgeway, 1981, 1984). The interaction between coping style and type of preoperative preparation has also been investigated (Cohen, 1975). The present study will contribute to the literature on the relationship between personality variables, effectiveness of the psychotherapeutic intervention, and recovery from surgery.

A substantial body of work has accumulated on the relationship between personality traits and the development of cancer (Cooper, 1984; Cox and Mackay, 1982; Fox, 1978, 1983; Greer, 1983; Greer and Watson, 1985; Grossarth-Maticek, 1980; Grossarth-Maticek et al., 1982, 1984, 1985; Wellisch and Yager, 1983), and of breast cancer in particular (Greer, 1976, 1979; Greer and Morris, 1975; Morris, 1980; Morris and Greer, 1982; Morris et al., 1981; Pettingale et al., 1984; Watson et al., 1984; Wirsching et al., 1982, 1985). The Courtauld Emotional Control Scale (Watson and Greer, 1983a, b) is now widely used, and the present study will contribute to the literature on patterns of emotional suppression and breast cancer.

The assessment of anxiety and depression in hospitalized populations presents psychometric problems. Self-report and interview measures correct for biases inherent in each when used alone, and both are included in the present study. The newly developed Hospital Anxiety and Depression Scale (Zigmond and Snaith, 1983) may be a more appropriate self-report measure for hospitalized patients than the General Health Questionnaire (Goldberg, 1978) although this needs to be demonstrated. The present study will allow for a comparison of the HADS and the GHQ in a population of surgical patients.

Streltzer and Leigh (1978) discuss the usefulness of a preoperative psychotherapeutic interview with surgical patients, adding that the most valuable approach could well be training surgeons to perform such interviews themselves. This has been accomplished in the present study. Our psychotherapeutic intervention is similar to interviews described in the liaison psychiatry literature (Lazarus and Hagens, 1968; Streltzer and Leigh, 1978; Viederman and Perry, 1980; Worden and Weisman, 1984). Background data for the psychotherapeutic intervention are gathered from the structured preoperative interview administered by a clinical psychologist.

Several recent studies of doctor-patient interaction and individual psychotherapy have employed Stiles' Verbal Response Modes (Stiles, 1978, 1978–1979, 1979). The scale provides a quantitative measure of psychotherapeutic responses such as reflection of feelings, interpretation, and acknowledgment. Categories also exist for self-disclosure, questions, confirmation, advisement, and edification [the giving of information]. In the present study we will be able to specify, from coded transcripts, what the surgeon is doing that is psychotherapeutic, and the nature of patients' responses. We will also be able to quantify the distinction between the psychotherapeutic intervention and the placebo attention control.

The purposes of the present study are five in number.

1. To assess the effectiveness of a programme of preoperative psychological preparation with mastectomy patients, using a structured interview and a 30-minute preoperative psychotherapeutic intervention. Two distinct but related objectives are involved: (a) to demonstrate the value of a preoperative brief psychotherapeutic intervention, and (b) to assess its value with a group of patients awaiting mastectomy. The emphasis in previous studies has been on *postoperative* intervention with mastectomy patients.

2. To assess the relationship between certain patient variables and psychological morbidity at follow-up. These variables include the impact of the diagnosis of cancer; health locus of control; anxiety and depression; emotional suppression; coping style; patients' beliefs about the cause of the illness; social support; stressful life events, and the meaning of the current illness in the context of the patient's life situation. If possible, to demonstrate any interactions between psychological variables and effectiveness of the psychotherapeutic intervention.

3. To contribute to the literature on psychological characteristics of breast cancer patients using the Courtauld Emotional Control Scale, and to compare the effectiveness of the Hospital Anxiety and Depression Scale and the General Health Questionnaire in the assessment of anxiety and depression in this patient population.

4. To demonstrate that with adequate training, a consultant surgeon can provide supportive psychological care for patients in a 30-min preoperative psychotherapeutic intervention. To our knowledge, our study is unique in this respect.

5. To specify the nature of the interaction between surgeon and patient in the brief psychotherapeutic intervention, using Stiles' Verbal Response Modes.

METHODS

The research began in March 1985 and is continuing at the present time. Patients eligible for inclusion in the study are admitted for either mastectomy or sector mastectomy under the care of any of the six consultant general surgeons at the Walsgrave Hospital. Patients awaiting excision biopsy and those with demonstrated benign diagnoses are not included. Occasionally patients are missed during the investigators' holidays or as a result of administrative errors. Twenty such patients have been missed thus far over a 21 month period. It is hoped eventually to include 200–250 patients in this study. This number will allow us to explore any interactions between psychological variables and response to the intervention. At the time of writing (November 1986), 103 patients are involved in the study, and some follow-up data are available on approximately 85 of these.

Patients are randomly assigned to one of four conditions:

(A) preoperative interview + brief psychotherapeutic intervention;
(B) preoperative interview + an equivalent amount of time spent chatting about unrelated matters (placebo attention control);
(C) preoperative interview only;
(D) routine hospital care control.

A fifth group includes those patients who were approached to participate in the study, but who declined to take part. This group represents 23% of patients who were approached in hospital.

The "interview only" group was included to control for any psychotherapeutic effects which might be occurring as a result of the preoperative interview alone. This group was added after the project had been running for a year, by which time 66 patients had already been recruited. Numbers in this "interview only" group remain too small at the time of writing to report any meaningful statistical results. Some preliminary results are however available for the intervention, chat and control groups, as well as for those patients who declined.

For patients in the three experimental groups, a structured preoperative interview is conducted by a clinical psychologist (MVB) on the afternoon or evening prior to surgery. The psychologist introduces herself by name, but not by profession, and says, "I am working with one of the surgeons on the floor. We are doing a study on the kinds of thoughts and feelings people have before an operation. I wonder if you would be willing to talk to me about what you've been feeling". Informed written consent is then obtained from those patients who wish to participate.

The preoperative interview covers the following areas:
discovery of the breast lump and referral to a surgeon;
the patient's beliefs about the cause of the illness;
her initial response to the need for surgery;
her desire for information about the operation;
worries about disturbance in body image and partner's response;
social support and stressful life events;
extent of past regrets and optimism/pessimism about the future;
anxiety and depression;
psychiatric history, if any;
worries about the anaesthetic;
concerns about outcome of the surgery; and

any other concerns the patient wishes to raise prior to surgery. The expression of feelings is encouraged, and a reflection of feelings technique is used where appropriate. The psychologist ends the interview by offering the patient a summary of her expressed worries and concerns, including a summary of those coping processes which have been most helpful to her. No attempt is made to challenge any of the patient's defences or coping styles. The interviews average 45–60 min in length. A few very distressed patients require more time.

Patients in the three experimental groups complete preoperatively the Impact of Event Scale (Horowitz and Wilner, 1980), the Multidimensional Health Locus of Control Scale (Wallston and Wallston, 1978), the General Health Questionnaire (Goldberg, 1978), the Hospital Anxiety and Depression Scale (Zigmond and Snaith, 1983), the Courtauld Emotional Control Scale (Watson and Greer, 1983a, b) and a revision of the Billings — Moos coping scale (Billings and Moos, 1981; Steptoe, personal communication).

Patients in the "interview only" condition receive no further intervention. Patients in both the intervention and chat conditions are told that Mr Parker, a consultant surgeon, will be coming to talk with them later that evening for about 30 min. Patients in group A receive a 30-min brief psychotherapeutic session with the surgeon. Patients in group B have a 30-min general chat with him about topics unrelated to the illness and surgery.

The brief psychotherapeutic intervention continues the process begun in the preoperative interview, encouraging the patient to discuss her feelings about the illness and surgery using a reflection of feelings technique in the Rogerian tradition of nondirective psychotherapy (Rogers, 1951, 1967). Information gathered from the preoperative interview is given to the surgeon in summary form so that he can provide a reflection to the patient of what he knows of her concerns. He spends 30-mins with her exploring her feelings about the surgery and illness in the context of her life situation. These interventions are audiotaped.

In the attention placebo control group, the surgeon spends 30-min chatting to the patient about unrelated matters, such as how long she has lived in Coventry, where she likes to go on holiday, how many children she has, what her hobbies are, and so on. No attempt is made to reflect feelings or explore the wider meaning of the illness. These friendly "chats" are also audiotaped.

Tapes of the interventions and chats are transcribed and then scored by three coders trained by the author of the Verbal Response Modes scoring system. These data will be reported in detail at a later time, but our preliminary impression is that there is a highly significant difference between interventions and chats. In the intervention, the surgeon gives many responses scored as reflection and acknowledgment. For example,

"You seem to be much more worried about the presence of the cancer than about the loss of the breast", is a reflection of the patient's feelings. "Um hm"'s and "Uh huh"'s (scored as acknowledgements) are used to encourage the patient to disclose more of what she is feeling. In response to the surgeon's reflective technique, patients in the intervention engage in significantly more disclosure of their feelings than the patients in the "chat" group.

A Recovery Index is calculated for all patients, including those who were approached but who declined to be interviewed. The Recovery Index includes both physical and psychological measures of adjustment to surgery and is obtained by taking the arithmetic sum of (a) postoperative days in hospital, (b) pain and sleep medications, (c) medical complications, and (d) negative psychological reactions noted by nursing staff (Cohen, 1975). Temperature, pulse and blood pressure charts are also retained, but these data have not yet been analyzed.

On the mastectomy patient's fourth postoperative day, a trained ward nurse or psychology technician readministers the anxiety and depression items from the preoperative interview. For those patients undergoing only sector mastectomy, the postoperative assessment is completed as early as postoperative day 2, immediately prior to discharge from hospital. At this time the patient also completes a postoperative Hospital Anxiety and Depression Scale.

Three months after surgery, a member of the Coventry Mastectomy Association telephones patients in all the groups (intervention, chat, interview only, and routine hospital care control) to arrange a brief interview on the patient's overall adjustment. Patients in the control group are told that the hospital is conducting a survey to see how patients feel as they recover from operations. Patients in the three experimental groups recall being seen in hospital prior to surgery, and are told that their progress is being followed at 3 months. Approximately ten women from the Coventry Mastectomy Association have been involved in these 3-month follow-up visits.

The Mastectomy Association worker sees the patient in her home for the interview, which covers the following areas: ability to cope with household chores, resumption of social activities, return to work (where applicable), feelings about the prosthesis, any problems with bras or clothing, any upset in looking at the scar, and any problems or worries about the future. The worker then asks the patient to complete and return the confidential postal questionnaire which includes a Hospital Anxiety and Depression Scale, the General Health Questionnaire Severe Depression Scale, and questions about the partner's response. In exceptional circumstances a 3-month interview is conducted by the clinical psychologist who saw the patient in hospital. Very occasionally an interview is carried out on the telephone, but the vast majority of the interviews are conducted by members of the Mastectomy Association in a domiciliary visit. Personnel other than the investigator are employed in the 4-day and 3-month outcome assessments wherever possible, in order to control for possible demand characteristics of the situation.

The psychologist follows up all patients at 1 year in a structured interview in the patient's home. This interview repeats the measures used at 3 months in addition to the patient's reactions to any recurrence, further surgery, radiotherapy, and chemotherapy. Anxiety and depression items from the preoperative interview are repeated. As yet, only about 40 patients have been assessed at 1 year, too small a sample for meaningful results to be reported at the present time.

The preoperative interviews are being coded for a number of relevant psychological variables:

1. Manuals have been developed for coding *coping style*, using both the Billings and Moos (1981) system [avoidant, cognitive and behavioural coping] and the Greer et al., (1979) system [denial, fighting spirit, stoic acceptance and helplessness/hopelessness]. A manual for the coding of *denial* has also been developed, based on a revision of the Hackett and Cassem (1974) scale for assessing denial in coronary patients. These coping and denial data will be reported at a later time (Burton and Simon, in preparation).

2. A revision of the manual for the *Leeds Attributional Coding System* (Stratton et al., 1986) has been developed which is applicable to cancer patients, and which allows for the coding of patients' attributions about the cause of the cancer along five dimensions; stable/unstable, global/specific, internal/external, personal/universal and controllable/uncontrollable (Burton and Hotson, in preparation). Attributional data obtained in this way may be correlated with locus of control, depression, and outcome measures at 3 months and 1 year. These results will be reported at a later time.

3. A manual has been developed for the scoring of *stressful life events*, yielding scores for (1) life events in the past 12 months; (2) more remote events; and (3) an overall stressful life events score. Stressful life events are scored 0 (no stressful events), 1 (low stress), 2 (moderate stress) and 3 (high stress). (Burton and Bailey, in preparation).

4. Patients who worry more about the anaesthetic than about the cancer and the disfigurement are an interesting group. A summated score for worries about the anaesthetic can be obtained from the interview, and this score correlated with the patient's preference for focusing on short-term rather than long-term worries and concerns. This coping style may also have implications for adjustment at 3 months and 1 year (Burton and Elcombe, in preparation).

TABLE 1. DEMOGRAPHIC VARIABLES AND BASIC MEDICAL DATA

Marital Status			
married	60%	widow, single, sep/div	41%
Age (means age 61 years)			
under 60	42%	over 60	58%
Social Class			
classes I, II	28%	classes III, IV and V	72%
Previous operations (mean 1.4)			
zero to 2	81.6%	3 and over	18.4%
Previous significant illness (mean 2.4)			
zero to 2	60%	3 and over	40%
Procedure			
sector mastectomy	43%	simple mastecomy	57%
Tumour, Nodes and Metastases (TNM)			
Stage I	8%	Stage II	50%
Stage III	40%	Stage IV	2%

RESULTS

Demographic variables and basic medical data

Demographic variables and basic medical data for the sample are shown in Table 1. There were no significant differences on any of these variables among patients in the four randomly assigned groups. Patients in the group who declined to participate varied from patients in the four randomly assigned groups only in that they tended to be older: 82.6% were over 60 compared to 66% in the randomly assigned groups.

Twelve patients received a benign histological diagnosis following their surgery. Of these, three had received a malignant diagnosis at previous surgery or biopsy. The incidence of benign histology did not differ significantly among the four randomly assigned groups.

Preoperative questionnaire data

Results of four preoperative questionnaires are shown in Table 2. Patients in the three experimental groups did not differ on any of these measures.

Patient scores on the Impact of Event Scale were similar to those recorded among patients suffering from stress response syndromes. Both the Hospital Anxiety and Depression Scale and the General Health Questionnaire detected a high incidence of preoperative anxiety and/or depression. These results will be discussed in more detail below.

Judging from scores on the Courtauld Emotional Control Scale, patients in the present study appear to suppress negative emotions to an even greater extent than previously reported populations of breast cancer

TABLE 2. MEAN SCORES ON FOUR PREOPERATIVE QUESTIONNAIRES. N = 66 PATIENTS

Impact of event scale	Avoidance 18.6	Intrusion 16.4	Total 35.0	
General health questionnaire				Total 5.2
Hospital Anxiety and depression scale		Anxiety 7.2	Depression 3.6	
Courtauld emotional control scale	Anger 17.9	Depression 19.2	Anxiety 19.0	Total 65.1

patients. Further work will investigate the relationship between emotional suppression, denial and avoidant coping. These three terms have been used almost interchangeably in some reported work. Our preliminary impression is that distinctions can be made among these variables (Burton and Simon, in preparation).

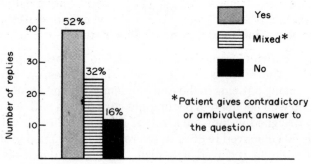

FIG. 1. DO YOU FEEL THAT YOU HAVE ENOUGH INFORMATION ABOUT YOUR OPERATION?

Preoperative interview data

Most of these data will be presented at a later date. Some initial findings can however be reported here.

Delay in presenting for treatment. Delay varied from a few days to 6 years. Sixty-six per cent consulted a doctor within a 3-month period. Thirty-four per cent delayed more than 3 months in seeking advice. Further work is planned to investigate the relationship between delay and other variables such as coping style.

Desire for information. Most patients expressed satisfaction with the information they had received, or gave an ambivalent reply when asked if they wished to be given any further information. A very small group gave an unambivalently negative reply to the question, "Do you feel that you have enough information about your operation?" (Fig 1).

Stressful life events. Our life stress measures have been developed in the tradition of the Brown and Harris (1978) model of contextual threat.

TABLE 3. STRESSFUL LIFE EVENTS

	Preceding 12 months	More remote stress	Overall score
Zero stressful life events	10.6%	1.5%	0%
Low stress	25.7%	24.3%	31.9%
Moderate stress	31.8%	25.7%	28.8%
Severe stress	31.8%	48.8%	29.4%

The incidence of stressful life events is shown in Table 3. It is noteworthy that 63.6% reported life stress in the preceding year which was scored as moderate to severe; 74.1% described moderate to severe life stress more remotely; and 58.2% experienced moderate to severe overall life stress (a composite measure taking into account both recent and remote stress).

Social support. Patients were asked about support from their husbands, family, friends, and religious groups. Specifically, they were asked whether they had been able to discuss their feelings about the operation with husband, family, friends or vicar. No sources of social support was reported by 11.9%; 21% one source; 35.5% two sources; 27.6% three sources; and 4% four sources.

Nature of preoperative anxiety. Patients were asked, "When you think about the operation you are going to have tomorrow, what are you most worried or concerned about?". Forty-four per cent were most preoccuped with immediate, short-term worries about the anaesthetic, going to theatre, needles, drips, and postoperative pain (Fig. 2). Twenty-one per cent were most concerned about the success of the surgery and

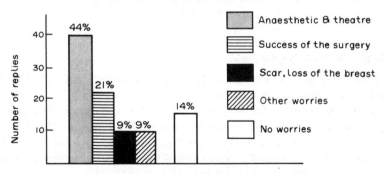

FIG. 2. WHEN YOU THINK ABOUT THE OPERATION YOU ARE GOING TO HAVE TOMORROW, WHAT ARE YOU MOST WORRIED OR CONCERNED ABOUT?

possible spread of the cancer; 9% were most worried about the scar or loss of the breast; and 9% were worried about other matters such as husband's reaction, worry about other people in the family, and ability to look after oneself and do things one enjoys. Fourteen per cent were not worried, and were unable to express any concerns when the follow-up question was asked, "Do you have any concerns about it at all?"

Screening for psychological distress. The General Health Questionnaire and the Hospital Anxiety and Depression Scale agreed on 83% of those cases which were identified by paper-and-pencil tests. In six instances there was disagreement, the GHQ tending to identify a case which the HADS missed twice as often ($n = 4$) as the HADS identified a case missed by the GHQ ($n = 2$).

Sometimes both the standardized interview measures of anxiety and depression and the questionnaire measures failed to reflect the patient's distress about her impending surgery. Only the clinical summary identified the patient's anxiety. Many of these cases carried the clinical summary, "Very anxious but denying", and despite the layers of denial, these patients were judged able to profit from a psychotherapeutic exploration of feelings.

The screening question in the present study was whether it is possible to identify those women sufficiently distressed to profit from preoperative intervention. Our concept of caseness is thus broader than the identification of depressive illness and/or anxiety state. We shall refer to these patients as the "worried" group. This group includes not only patients with substantial anxiety and/or depression but others with distress that does not reach PSE or HADS/GHQ threshold. The unworried women are a small but identifiable group. When they are offered preoperative psychotherapeutic interventions, there are no feelings of concern for the surgeon to reflect:

"So you're not worried about the disfigurement." – "No."

"And you're not particularly worried about the cancer." – "No."

"And you have no particular worries about the anaesthetic." – "No!"

and so on. These women were not in need of exploring worries, and intervention was therefore unnecessary. Eighteen per cent ($n = 14$) of the present sample interviewed ($n = 76$) were not worried or concerned about either the illness or the surgery.

Among the remaining 82%, 49% were suffering from significant anxiety or depression, using the criteria of the modified PSE interview schedule and confirmed by the HADS and/or the GHQ, and the clinical impression of the interviewer. An additional 16% reached caseness criterion on either the HADS or the GHQ, confirmed by the interviewer's clinical impression. A further 17% were judged sufficiently distressed at interview to profit from intervention. In these cases neither the PSE nor the HADS/GHQ measures had identified the patient as a case, but distress was evident at interview (Fig. 3).

"Worry" was significantly related to age (ANOVA, $f = 7.767$, $p < .0068$), marital status (Chi^2 = 4.422, $p < 0.0333$) and overall stressful life events (Krushal-Wallis, $H = 4.709$, $p < 0.0281$). Women under 60,

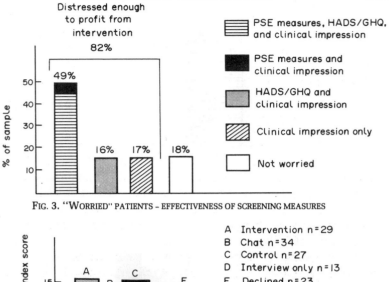

FIG. 3. "WORRIED" PATIENTS – EFFECTIVENESS OF SCREENING MEASURES

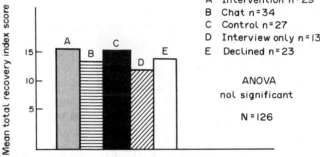

FIG. 4. RECOVERY INDEX

married women and women with significant overall stressful life event scores were more likely to be worried than women over 60, women on their own, and women without significant overall stressful life events. There were no significant differences among experimental groups on PSE interview measures of anxiety and depression, HADS caseness, "worry", social support or stressful life events.

Outcome measures: 1. Recovery Index data

No significant differences were found between experimental groups on the Recovery Index (Fig. 4).

Procedure significantly predicted Recovery Index scores (ANOVA, $f = 24.355$, $P < 0.0001$): patients undergoing simple mastectomy had significantly higher Recovery Index scores than women undergoing sector mastectomies.

Outcome data: 2. 3-month interview distress scores

Differences in overall functioning were identifiable between groups at 3 months (Fig. 5). An analysis of variance of 3-month interview distress

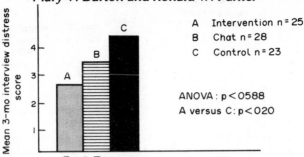

A   Intervention n = 25
B   Chat n = 28
C   Control n = 23

ANOVA : p < 0588
A versus C : p < 020

FIG. 5. THREE-MONTH INTERVIEW SCORE

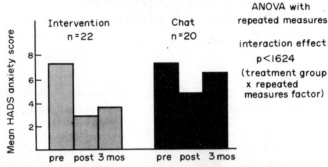

ANOVA with repeated measures

interaction effect
p < 1624
(treatment group x repeated measures factor)

FIG. 6. HADS ANXIETY SCORES: PREOPERATIVELY, POST
OPERATIVELY AND AT 3 MONTHS

scores approaches significance ($f = 2.917$, P < 0.0588), and there was a statistically significant difference in distress at interview between interventions and controls (P = < 0.02).

Outcome measures: 3. HADS anxiety scores over time

The pattern of HADS anxiety over time shows significant differences between the intervention and chat groups (Fig. 6). Both groups experience a decrease in anxiety during the immediate postoperative period. Anxiety at 3 months has however risen to higher levels among patients in the chat group than among those in the intervention group. An analysis of variance with repeated measures approaches significance for an interaction between the grouping factor and the repeated measures factor ($f = 1.847$, P < 0.1624).

When only those patients considered "worried" are included in the analysis, there is a statistically significant treatment effect ($f = 4.854$, P < 0.332, Fig 7).

No such treatment effect appears in HADS depression scores over time (Fig. 8).

"Worry" was a significant predictor of 3-month HADS anxiety (ANOVA, $f = 11.432$, P < 0.0017) and 3-month HADS depression ($f =$

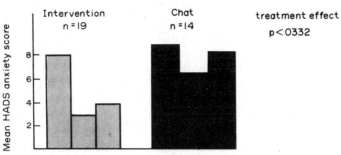

FIG. 7. HADS ANXIETY SCORES: PREOPERATIVELY, POST OPERATIVELY
AND AT
3 MONTHS — "WORRIED" PATIENTS ONLY

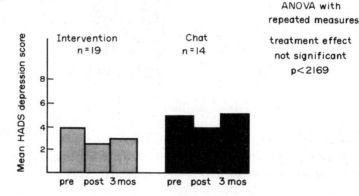

FIG. 8. HADS DEPRESSION SCORES: PREOPERATIVELY, POSTOPERATIVELY
AND AT 3 MONTHS — "WORRIED" PATIENTS ONLY

4.004, P <0.0473). HADS caseness was a significant predictor of 3-month distress (f = 12.726, P <0.0011), 3-month HADS anxiety (f = 18.296, P <0.0002) and 3-month HADS depression (f = 13.571, P <0.0008). Those found to be distressed in hospital were thus likely to evidence more distress at 3 months than those found to have no worries or concerns preoperatively.

Two other predictor variables, equally distributed among experimental groups, were shown to affect HADS scores at 3 months. Overall stressful life events predicted HADS anxiety (f = 4.530, P <0.0149) and HADS depression (f = 3.502, P <0.0360) scores. Women with more severe life events had higher scores on the HADS at 3 months.

Procedure was also found to be a significant predictor variable of HADS anxiety (f = 6.848, P <0.0109) and depression (f = 6.030, P <0.0162) at 3 months. Women undergoing sector mastectomy scored higher on both HADS anxiety and HADS depression at 3 months than women who had undergone the more extensive simple mastectomy. The relative importance of these and other potentially meaningful variables in predicting outcome at 3 months and 1 year will eventually be tested in a regression analysis. Our limited sample size at the present time would make such an analysis statistically unreliable at this stage.

DISCUSSION

Avoidance subscores on the Impact of Event Scale (Table 2) are very similar to published scores of patients suffering from stress response syndromes (Horowitz et al., 1979): Avoidance 18.2; Intrusion 21.4 and Total 39.5 among stress response syndrome patients, compared to scores in the present sample of 18.6, 16.4 and 35.0 respectively.

Published scores of breast cancer patients on the Courtauld Emotional Control Scale (Watson and Greer, 1983b) are slightly lower than scores in the present sample: Anger 16.8, Depression 18.1, Anxiety 17.9 and Total 52.6. Our patients' scores were 17.9, 19.0 and 56.1 respectively. Thus patients in our study appear to suppress negative emotions to an even greater extent than previously reported breast cancer patients.

The incidence of depressive illness and/or anxiety state in our sample is higher than that reported in a well-known study of mastectomy patients in the U.K. Maguire et al. (1978) reported a 27% incidence of moderate or severe anxiety, a 16% incidence of moderate or severe depression, and overall, a 31% incidence of moderate or severe anxiety or depression or both in women awaiting mastectomy. In our study there was a 47% incidence of significant anxiety, a 28% incidence of significant depression, and overall, a 49% incidence of significant anxiety or depression, using PSE criteria. It is possible that our figures are higher because a substantial number of patients who were approached (23%) declined to participate in the study. Many of these insisted when approached that they were not worried. There may therefore be some self-selection in the direction of more distressed women electing to participate in the study, thus inflating somewhat our figures for PSE caseness. Our patient population includes both mastectomy and sector mastectomy patients, whereas Maguire studied mastectomy patients exclusively. Preoperative HADS depression scores were on average twice as high among patients awaiting sector mastectomies than among those awaiting mastectomy $(f = 6.927, P < 0.0102)$. Preoperative HADS anxiety scores were also higher among those awaiting sector mastectomy, although this relationship did not reach the level of statistical significance $(f = 2.352, P < 0.1259)$. If these findings are confirmed with larger samples, our higher levels of anxiety and depression on PSE criteria may be in part a function of the number of sector mastectomies in our sample.

It has been estimated that between 35 and 50% of cancer patients delay seeking medical advice for more than 3 months (Antonovsky and Hartman, 1974). In our sample, 34% delayed for this length of time before consulting a doctor, close to the lower limit of the range established in other studies.

There is now a very substantial literature on patient dissatisfaction with information given to them in hospital (Ley, 1982). The fact that only 16% said clearly that they wished to have more information is perhaps surprising in this context. A very substantial number of women who replied "yes" to the question about information, or gave a mixed response, said such things as "I'd rather not know"; "I'm not sure I want all the questions answered now"; "The less I know about it the better"; "What if don't know won't hurt me" or "Ignorance is bliss". This lack of desire to know about the operation may be related to coping styles of avoidance or denial. It may also be related to a pattern of suppression of negative thoughts or emotions as reflected in high CECS scores. An investigation of the relationship between desire for information, personality variables and demographic variables such as social class will be reported at a later time. It is also possible that increased attention to breast cancer in the media has provided many patients with information about their illness prior to hospitalization; or that surgeons and nursing staff, aware of the increased public interest in breast cancer and mastectomy, are taking greater care to explain the procedure carefully to patients.

Studies of the relationship between stressful life events and breast cancer have been equivocal (Ray and Baum, 1985). We have found a high level of stressful life events in our population, but it is difficult to compare our findings with those of existing studies because (a) we have not investigated a control group of patients with benign breast disease; and (b) several recent existing studies in this area have used questionnaire measures such as the Schedule of Recent Experiences (Holmes and Rahe, 1967). For methodological reasons we have chosen to use an interview measure and our manual for scoring stressful events has been developed within the framework of the "contextual threat" of the life event to the patient (Brown and Harris, 1978). Ray and Baum (1985) observe that the use of paper-and-pencil measures is probably less sensitive to the personal meaning of events than interview measures, and many writers suggest that questionnaires have now become discredited as life event indices. We may thus be better able to discover the meaning of life events to the patient in our interview protocol than investigators who rely on questionnaire measures alone, predisposing us perhaps to discover higher frequencies of life stress. Relationships among stressful life events, social support, coping style, personality variables, caseness and surgical procedure will be reported at a later time. At the present time, it is clear that overall stressful life event scores significantly affect 3-month HADS anxiety and depression, in the direction that would be predicted.

The salience of stressful life events also extends to implications for surgical practice. From an ongoing research project on surgeons' attitudes towards psychological aspects of surgery (Burton, in preparation), it is clear that few surgeons enquire about the occurrence of stressful life events in their assessment of the patient prior to surgery. The current study suggests that this may be an important omission, as the impact of stressful life events appears to extend well into the postoperative period.

Social support is frequently cited as a moderator of the stress of diagnosis and surgery (Bloom, 1982). Several recent studies have challenged the traditional view of social support as a buffer of stress, suggesting that social support might constitute a stress in itself (Dunkel-Schetter and Wortman, 1982; Fiore et al., 1983). "Worried" women in the present study were significantly more likely to be married. It is possible that some of this effect is due to the stress of a larger social network on the patient. It is also possible that higher recovery index scores in the present sample among married women could reflect the increased number of family worries these women experience, compared to single or widowed women. Social support was among the variables that predicted 3-month HADS depression, although it was a complicated relationship. The highest levels of depression were found in the six women with no sources of social support. However, as sources of social support increased from 1 to 4, there was a trend in the direction of more depression with increasing availability of social support. It is also possible that women suffering more depression use social support to a greater extent than non-depressed women. These findings need to be confirmed with larger samples, taking into account the quality of the patient's relationships and any interactions with other variables such as age. However, it may be that for some women, stress is multiplied when there are worries about husband's response and children's welfare. Social support in these instances may constitute an additional source of stress rather than a buffer of stress.

Screening of cancer patients for psychotherapeutic interventions has received considerable attention recently (Worden and Weisman, 1980; Worden, 1983). Recent studies of the incidence of psychological distress in cancer patients have employed concurrently interview measures such as the Present State Examination and questionnaire measures (Fallowfield et al., 1986). Most screening procedures have involved some combination of interview and questionnaire measures and in this respect the present study is consistent with previous work. One noteworthy feature of our findings is the number of worried patients missed by formal methods such as the PSE and the HADS or GHQ. Some of those patients who are "worried but denying" are discovered only at interview. It may be possible to identify some subset of interview questions which would reliably identify those women who could profit from intervention. This screening question will be addressed as we gather data on a larger number of patients.

Our lack of treatment effect on Recovery Index is consistent with two recent critiques of recovery as an outcome measure of preoperative interventions (Johnston, 1984; Viney et al., 1985). Recovery Index scores are calculated from a number of subscores, among them number of days in hospital. Administrative policy with regard to bed allocation may substantively affect number of days in hospital, as may the presence or absence of social support. In the present study, discharge was delayed on a number of occasions when patients' social problems were discovered belatedly and arrangements for convalescence had to be made because the patient was unable to return to a council flat where she had little or no support. One recent study suggested that the variable with best predictive power of recovery was severity of illness and extent of surgery (Viney et al., 1985). This finding has been confirmed in the present study. Recovery Index scores in the mastectomy group were, on average, twice as high as those of sector mastectomy patients.

The finding of greater anxiety and depression at 3 months in sector mastectomy patients than in mastectomy patients confirms the findings of a recent study (Fallowfield et al., 1986). Postoperatively, there was a 38% incidence of anxiety state, depressive illness or both in sector mastectomy patients as opposed to 33% among mastectomy patients in a comparable study employing virtually the same measure used in the present study. We have also found a higher level of anxiety and/or depression among sector mastectomy patients, which suggests that concern about cancer recurrence may account for more postoperative concern than the loss of the breast. Women undergoing sector mastectomy may have more worries about recurrence than those undergoing mastectomy, though this hypothesis must be confirmed by a more detailed analysis of the 3-month and 1-year data with larger samples.

The significant treatment effect is consistent with a number of studies which have demonstrated the effectiveness of psychosocial support and counselling in patients' psychological adjustment to breast cancer and mastectomy (Gordon et al., 1980; Maguire et al., 1980a, 1983; Morganstern et al., 1984; Pfefferbaum et al., 1977–1978; Watson, 1983; Wellisch, 1984). The abrupt decline in anxiety postoperatively has been noted in previous studies of pre- and post-operative anxiety levels

(Spielberger *et al.*, 1973). However, anxiety is seen to increase at 3 months among "chat" patients while remaining low in intervention patients. The effect is most apparent when only "worried" women are offered the extra support. Some benefit is nevertheless derived by those women not in need of intervention (Sobel and Worden, 1982).

It would thus appear that a 30-min intervention focused on the patient's feelings is superior to a friendly, nontherapeutic chat in affecting anxiety at 3 months. Future work will be able to specify precisely the difference between the interventions and chats in terms of Verbal Response Modes. These findings have relevance for doctor–patient communication more generally: they suggest that the affable, friendly approach many doctors employ in support of their patients is less effective in moderating psychological distress than reflection of feelings, a technique which can be relatively easily learnt by doctors with the motivation to do so.

Not all members of the medical or surgical profession are, however, so motivated. In our initial research design, house surgeons at the Walsgrave Hospital were approached with respect to doing the preoperative interviews, psychotherapeutic interventions and chats under the supervision of a clinical psychologist. It was felt that this experience would be valuable to the junior doctors as part of their training. Their response revealed a pronounced lack of interest in the psychosocial dimension of illness among at least one small sample of recent medical school graduates. One house surgeon, for example, replied: "Why should I learn to talk to patients about their feelings? How could that possibly help me in my medical career?"

When four of the six house surgeons refused to be involved in the project, the investigators decided to carry out the project themselves, the clinical psychologist to do the preoperative interviews and the consultant surgeon to do the chats and interventions.

As a result of participating in this research project, the surgeon has found that various aspects of his clinical work have been affected. History-taking has been improved, partly by engaging with the patient's feelings and putting them at their ease; patients think more clearly that way. Inquiry into areas of the history not normally undertaken by clinicians has brought much useful material into view relevant to the diagnosis. There is increased understanding of the complexity of the human being and the wide range of feelings which may produce the final common pathway of a symptom, e.g,. pain in the abdomen. This has reduced the anger and frustration in the surgeon when no physical cause is found for the symptom, on investigation. Thus the frequency of the pejorative diagnosis, "neurotic patient", made in anger, is reduced. This helps the clinician to think more clearly and to keep options open. Referral of such a patient for psychiatric interview to help in the diagnosis has generally been found to be unhelpful, as a psychiatrist will usually report that the patient does not suffer from a psychiatric illness. Similarly, when examining a patient, it is much more helpful to have communicated to the patient that the clinician understands his or her feelings. For instance, the simple examination of sigmoidoscopy in outpatients, when carried out sympathetically, enables a much more extensive examination to take place than when the patient is intimidated by ten inches of cold steel being waved unfeelingly in his direction. The same is true of many other physical examinations.

Taking this approach with patients has not altered surgical decision-making in any detectable way. It could be argued that exploring patients' feelings increases the stress on the surgeon. However, our experience has been that once one is aware of a patient's feelings, it becomes stressful not to discuss them.

Having reached a diagnosis, the understanding of a patient's feelings will enable a much more sympathetic and relevant discussion to take place. Sometimes this will involve the discussion of a large and mutilating operation and its consequences, or a painful investigation. Or it may facilitate a more confident exploration of the patient's feelings and anxieties, on those occasions when the physical problem is essentially a byproduct of stress. The process of engaging with patients' feelings has also been of help in dealing with the dying patient and his or her relatives. Awareness of patients' and relatives' feelings and worries has been helpful in the sphere of management. It has been a constant concern to "humanize" the face of the health service, and to improve the quality of service provided. Patients often find their experience frightening and intimidating, and they often accuse the health service of being unresponsive to their needs. An understanding of the feelings patients experience in coming to hospital has frequently informed discussions on the district team and hopefully will result in more sympathetic patient care.

In our experience, this approach has widened the diagnostic window and improved confidence in dealing with the patient's psychosocial needs. It is important that medical schools improve training in this area, and that this process of learning continue in teaching hospitals.

ACKNOWLEDGEMENTS

This research has been supported since July 1986 by a grant from the Cancer Research Campaign.

REFERENCES

Anderson, K. O. and Masur, F.T. (1983) Psychological preparation for invasive medical and dental procedures. *J. Behav. Med.* **6**, 1–40.

Antonovsky, A. and Hartman, M.A. (1974) Delay in the detection of cancer: A review of the literature. *Health Educ. Monogr.* **2**, 98-128.

Asken, M. J. (1975) Psychoemotional aspects of mastectomy: A review of recent literature. *Am. J. Psychiat.* **132**, 56-59.

Baider, L., Amikam, J. C. and De-Nour, A. K. (1984 Time-limited thematic group with post-mastectomy patients. *J. Psychosom. Res.* **28**, 323-330.

Baum, M. and Jones, E. (1979) Counselling removes patients' fear. *Nurs. Mirror* **48**, 39-41.

Beckmann, J., Blichert-Toft, J. and Johansen, L. (1983) Psychological effects of mastectomy. *Dan. Med. Bull.* **30**, 7-10.

Billings, A. G. and Moos, R. H. (1981) The role of coping responses and social resources in attenuating the stress of life events. *J. Behav. Med.* **4**, 139-157.

Blake, S. (1984) Group therapy with breast cancer patients. In *Psychological Aspects of Cancer* Watson M. and Morris T., eds., pp. 93-98. Pergamon Press, Oxford.

Bloom, J. R. (1982) Social support, accommodation to stress, and adjustment to breast cancer. *Soc. Sci. Med.* **16**, 1329-1338.

Bloom, J. R. Ross, R. D. and Burnell, G. (1978) The effect of social support on patient adjustment after breast surgery. *Patient Counsel. Health Educ.* **1**, 50-59.

Brown, G. W. and Harris, T. (1978) *The Social Origins of Depression.* Tavistock, London.

Burton, M. V. (in preparation) Psychological aspects of surgery: Surgeons' attitudes. Presented at "The Doctor, The Patient, The Illness", University of Durham, July 1986. Unpublished manuscript.

Burton, M. V. and Bailey, D. (in preparation) Stressful life events in breast cancer patients.

Burton, M. V. and Elcombe, S. (in preparation) Short-term and long-term worries in patients awaiting mastectomy.

Burton, M. V. and Hotson, S. (in preparation) Attributions about the cause of illness in breast cancer patients.

Burton, M. V. and Simon, D. (in preparation) Avoidant coping, denial and emotional suppression in mastectomy patients.

Christenson, D. N. (1983) Postmastectomy couple counselling: An outcome study of a structured treatment protocol. *J. Sex Marital Ther.* **9**, 266-275.

Cohen, F. (1975) Psychological preparation, coping and recovery from surgery. *Diss. Abs. Int.* **37**, 454B.

Cohen, F. and Lazarus, R. S. (1973) Active coping processes, coping dispositions, and recovery from surgery. *Psychosom. Med.* **35**, 375-389.

Cooper, C. L., ed. (1984) *Psychosocial Stress and Cancer.* Wiley, Chichester.

Cox, T. and Mackay, C. (1982) Psychosocial factors and psychophysiological mechanisms in the aetiology and development of cancers. *Soc. Sci. Med.* **16**, 381-396.

Devine, E. C. and Cook, T. D. (1983) A meta-analytic analysis of effects of psychoeducational interventions on length of postsurgical hospital stay. *Nurs. Res.* **32**, 267-274.

Dunkel-Schetter, C. and Wortman, C. B. (1982) The interpersonal dynamics of cancer: Problems in social relationships and their impact on the patient. In Friedman, H. S. and DiMatteo, M. R., eds, *Interpersonal Issues in Health Care*, Academic Press, New York.

Fallowfield, L. J., Baum, M. and Maguire, G. P. (1986) Effects of breast conservation on psychological morbidity associated with diagnosis and treatment of early breast cancer. *Br. Med. J.* **293**, 1331-1334.

Faulkner, A. and Maguire, P. (1984) Teaching ward nurses to monitor cancer patients. *Clin. Oncol.* **10**, 383-389.

Fiore, J., Becker J. and Coppel, D. B. (1983) Social network interactions: A buffer or a stress. *Am. J. Community Psychol.* **11**, 423-439.

Fox, B. H. (1978) Premorbid psychological factors as related to cancer incidence. *J. Behav. Med.* **1**, 45-133.

Fox, B. H. (1983) Current theory of psychogenic effects on cancer incidence and prognosis. *J. Psychosoc. Oncol.* **1**, 17-22.

Gerard, D. (1982) Sexual functioning after mastectomy: Life vs. lab. *J. Sex Marital Ther.* **8**, 305-315.

Gil, K. M. (1984) Coping effectively with invasive medical procedures: A descriptive model. *Clin. Psychol. Rev.* **4**, 339-362.

Goldberg, D. (1978) *Manual of the General Health Questionnaire.* NFER-Nelson, Windsor.

Goldberg, J. G., ed. (1981) *Pschotherapeutic Treatment of Cancer Patients.* Free Press, New York.

Gordon, W. A., Freidenbergs, I., Diller, L., Hibbard, M., Wolf, C., Levine, L. Lipkins, R. Ezrachi, O. and Lucido, D. (1980) Efficacy of psychosocial intervention with cancer patients. *J. Consult. Clin. Psychol.* **48**, 743–759.

Greer, S. (1976) Psychological correlates of breast cancer. In Stoll, B. ed., *Risk Factors in Breast Cancer* pp. 71–79. Heinemann, London.

Greer, S. (1979) Psychological attributes of women with breast cancer. *Cancer Detect. Prevent.* **2**, 289–294.

Greer, S. (1983) Cancer and the mind. *Br. J. Psychiat.* **143**, 535–543.

Greer, S. and Morris, T. (1975) Psychological attributes of women who develop breast cancer. A controlled study. *J. Psychosom. Res.* **19**, 147–153.

Greer, S. and Watson, M. (1985) Towards a psychobiological model of cancer: Psychological considerations. *Soc. Sci. Med.* **20**, 773–777.

Greer, S., Morris, T. and Pettingale, K. (1979) Psychological response to breast cancer: Effect on outcome. *Lancet*, 785–787.

Grossarth-Maticek, R. (1980) Psychosocial precursors of cancer and internal diseases. *Psychother. Psychosom.* **33**, 122–128.

Grossarth-Maticek, R., Siegrist, J. and Vetter, H. (1982) Interpersonal repression as a predictor of cancer. *Soc. Sci. Med.* **16**, 493–498.

Grossarth-Maticek, R., Frentzel-Beyne, R. and Becker, N. (1984) Cancer risks associated with life events and conflict solution. *Cancer Detect. Prevent.* **7**, 201–209.

Grossarth-Maticek, R., Bastiaans, J. and Kanazir, D. T. (1985) Psychosocial factors as strong predictors of mortality from cancer, ischaemic heart disease and stroke: The Yugoslav prospective study. *J. Psychosom. Res.* **29**, 167–176.

Hackett, T. P. and Cassem, N. H. (1974) Development of a quantitative rating scale to assess denial. *J. Psychosom. Res.* **18**, 93–100.

Holmes, T. H. Rahe, R. H. (1967) The social readjustment rating scale. *J. Psychosom. Res.* **11**, 219–255.

Horowitz, M. J. and Wilner, N. (1980) Life events, stress and coping. In *Aging in the 1980s: Psychological Issues* Poon, L. ed., pp. 363–374. Am. Psychological Association. Washington, DC.

Horowitz, M. J., Wilner, N. and Alvarez, W. (1979) Impact of Event Scale: A measure of subjective stress. *Psychosom. Med.* **41**, 209–218.

Jamison, K. R., Wellisch, D. K. and Pasnau, R. O. (1978) Psychosocial aspects of mastectomy I. The woman's perspective. *Am. J. Psychiat.* **135**, 432–436.

Jamison, K. R. Wellisch, D. K., Katz, R. L. and Pasnau, R. O. (1979) Phantom breast syndrome. *Arch. Surg.* **11**, 93–95.

Janis, I. (1983) Stress inoculation in health care: Theory and research. In *Stress Reduction and Prevention* Meichenbaum, D. and Jarenko, M.E., eds, pp. 67–99. Plenum: New York.

Johnston, M. (1984) Dimensions of recovery from surgery. *Int. Rev. Appl. Psychol.* **33**, 505–520.

Kendall, P. C. (1983) Stressful medical procedures: Cognitive-behavioral strategies for stress management and prevention. In *Stress Reduction and Prevention* Meichenbaum, D., Jarenko, M. E. eds, pp. 159–190. Plenum: New York.

Kleiman, M. A., Mantell, J. E. and Alexander, E. S. (1977) Rx for social death: The cancer patient as counsellor. *Community Ment. Health J.* **13**, 115–124.

Lazurus, H. R. and Hagens, J. H. (1968) Prevention of psychosis following open-heart surgery. *Am. J. Psychiat.* **124**, 1190–1195.

Ley, P. (1982) Giving information to patients. In *Social Psychology and Behavioral Medicine* Eiser, J. R. ed, pp. 339–371. Wiley, Chichester.

Lierman, L. (1982) Psychological preparation and supportive care for mastectomy patients. *West. J. Nurs. Res.* **4**, 13–19.

Lierman, L. (1984) Support for mastectomy: A clinical nursing research study, *Assoc. of Operating Room Nurs. J.* **39**, 1150–1157.

MacDonald, M. R. and Kuiper, N. A. (1983) Cognitive-behavioural preparations for surgery: Some theoretical and methodological concerns. *Clin. Psychol. Rev.* **3**, 27–39.

Maguire, G. P. (1984) Psychological intervention in women with breast cancer. In

Psychological Aspects of Cancer Watson, M., Morris T., eds, pp. 77-83. Pergamon Press, Oxford.

Maguire, G. P. Lee, E. G. Bevington, D. J. Kuchemann, C. S. Crabtree, R. J. and Cornell, C. E. (1978). Psychiatric problems in the first year after mastectomy. *Br. Med. J.* **1**, 963-965.

Maguire, G. P. Tait, A., Brooke, M. and Sellwood, R. (1980a) Emotional aspects of mastectomy: Planning a caring programme. *Nurs. Mirror* **150**, 35-37.

Maguire, G. P., Tait, A., Brooke, M., Thomas, C. and Sellwood, R. (1980b) The effects of counselling on the psychiatric morbidity associated with mastectomy. *Br. Med. J.* **281**, 1454-1456.

Maguire, G. P. Brooke, M. Tait, A., Thomas, C. and Sellwood, R. (1983) The effect of counselling on physical disability and social recovery after mastectomy. *Clin. Oncol.* **9**, 319-324.

Mathews, A. and Ridgeway, V. (1981) Personality and surgical recovery: A review. *Br. J. Clin. Psychol.* **20**, 243-260.

Mathews, A. and Ridgeway, V. (1984) Psychological preparation for surgery. In *Health Care and Human Behaviour*, Steptoe, A. and Mathews, A. eds, pp. 231-259. Academic Press, London.

Morganstern, H., Gellert, G. A., Walter, S. D., Ostfeld, A. M. and Siegel, B. S. (1984) The impact of a psychosocial support program on survival with breast cancer: The importance of selection bias in program evaluation. *J. Chronic Dis.* **37**, 273-282.

Morris, T. (1980) 'Type C' for cancer? Low trait anxiety in the pathogenesis of breast cancer. *Cancer Detect. Prevent.* **3**, 102.

Morris, T. and Greer, S. (1982) Psychological characteristics of women electing to attend a breast screening clinic. *Clin. Oncol.* **8**, 113-119.

Morris, T., Greer, S. and White, P. (1977) Psychological and social adjustment to mastectomy: A two year follow up study. *Cancer* **40**, 2381-2387.

Morris, T., Greer, S., Pettingale, K. W. and Watson, M. (1981) Patterns of expression of anger and their psychological correlates in women with breast cancer. *J. Psychosom. Res.* **25**, 111-117.

Mumford, E., Schlesinger, H. J. and Glass, G. V. (1982) The effect of psychological intervention on recovery from surgery and heart attacks: An analysis of the literature. *Am. J. Pub. Health* **72**, 141-151.

Pettingale, K. W., Watson, M. and Greer, S. (1984) The validity of emotional control as a trait in breast cancer patients. *J. Psychosoc. Oncol.* **2**, 21-30.

Pfefferbaum, B., Pasnau, R. O., Jamison, K. and Wellisch, D. K. (1977-1978) A comprehensive program of psychological care for mastectomy patients. *Int. J. Psychiat. Med.* **8**, 63-72.

Ray, C. (1977) Psychological implications of mastectomy. *Br. J. Soc. Clin. Psychol.* **16**, 373-377.

Ray, C. (1978) Adjustment to mastectomy: The psychological impact of disfigurement. In Brand, P. C. and vanKeep, P. A. eds, *Breast Cancer: Psychosocial Aspects of Early Detection and Treatment*, pp. 33-45. University Park Press: Baltimore.

Ray, C. and Baum, M. (1985) *Psychological Aspects of Early Breast Cancer*. Springer, New York.

Reading, A. E. (1979) The short term effects of psychological preparation for surgery. *Social Sci. Med.* **13**, 641-654.

Rogers, C. R. (1951) *Client-centered Therapy*. Houghton Mifflin, Boston.

Rogers, C. R. (1967) *The Therapeutic Relationship and Its Impact*. University of Wisconsin Press, Madison, Wisconsin.

Schwartz, M. D. (1977) An information and discussion program for women after mastectomy. *Arch. Surg.* **112**, 276-281.

Sobel, H. J. and Worden, J. W. (1982) *Helping Cancer Patients Cope: A Problem Solving Intervention Program for Health Care Professionals*. B.M.A. Audio Cassettes, Guilford Publications, New York.

Spiegel, D., Bloom, J. R. and Yalom, I. (1981) Group support for patients with metastatic cancer. *Arch. Gen. Psychiat.* **38**, 527-533.

Spielberger, C. D. Auerbach, S. M. Wadsworth, A. P. Dunn, T. M. and Taulbee, E. S. (1973) Emotional reactions to surgery. *J. Consult. Clin. Psychol.* **40**, 33-38.

Steptoe, A. (1985, personal communication) A revision of the Billings & Moos coping scale used in psychological study of coronary bypass patients.

Stiles, W. B. (1978) *Manual for a Taxonomy of Verbal Response Modes.* Institute for Research in Social Science, University of North Carolina, Chapel Hill.

Stiles, W. B. (1978-1979) Discourse analysis and the doctor-patient relationship. *Int. J. Psychiat. Med.* **9**, 263-273.

Stiles, W. B. (1979) Verbal response modes and psychotherapeutic technique. *Psychiatry* **42**, 49-62.

Stratton, P., Munton, T., Heard, D., Hanks, H. and Davidson, C. (1986) *Leeds Attributional Coding System (LACS) Manual.* Family Research Centre, Department of Psychology, University of Leeds. Unpublished manuscript.

Streltzer, J. and Leigh, H. (1978) Psychological preparation for surgery: The usefulness of a preoperative psychotherapeutic interview. *Hawaii Med. J.* **37**, 139-142.

Tait, A., Maguire, P., Faulkner, A., Brooke, M., Wilkinson, S., Thomson, L. and Sellwood, R. (1982) Improving communication skills: Standardized assessments may help nurses to detect psychiatric problems as they develop in mastectomy patients. *Nurs. Times* **78**, 2181-2184.

Tarrier, N. and Maguire, P. (1984) Treatment of psychological distress following mastectomy: An initial report. *Behav. Res. Ther.* **22**, 81-84.

Tarrier, N., Maguire, P. and Kincey, J. (1983) Locus of control and cognitive behaviour therapy with mastectomy patients: A pilot study. *Br. J. Med. Psychol.* **56**, 265-270.

Tierney, J. and Murrell, D. (1985) The Mastectomy Association. *Practitioner* **229**, 265-267.

Vachon, M. L. S., Lyall, W. A. L., Rogers, J., Cochrane, J. and Freeman, S. J. J. (1981-1982) The effectiveness of psychosocial support during post-surgical treatment of breast cancer. *Int. J. Psychiat. Med.* **11**, 365-372.

Viederman, M. and Perry, S. W. (1980) Use of psychodynamic life narrative in the treatment of depression in the physically ill. *Gen. Hosp. Psychiat.* **3**, 177-185.

Viney, L. L., Clarke, A. M. Bunn, T. A. and Benjamin, Y. N. (1985) The effect of a hospital-based counselling service on the physical recovery of surgical and medical patients. *Gen. Hosp. Psychiat.* **7**, 294-301.

Wallston, K. A. and Wallston, B. S. (1978) Development of the Multidimensional Health Locus of Control (MHLC) scales. *Health Educ. Monog.* **6**, 160-170.

Watson, M. (1983) Psychosocial intervention with cancer patients: A review. *Psychol. Med.* **13**, 839-846.

Watson, M. and Greer, S. (1983a) *A Preliminary Manual for the Courtauld Emotional Control Scale.* Faith Courtauld Unit, King's College Hospital: London. Unpublished report.

Watson, M. and Greer, S. (1983b) Development of a questionnaire measure of emotional control. *J. Psychosom. Res.* **27**, 299-305.

Watson, M., Pettingale, K. W. and Greer, S. (1984) Emotional control and autonomic arousal in breast cancer patients. *J. Psychosom. Res.* **28**, 467-474.

Wellisch, D. K. (1984) Implementation of psychosocial services in managing emotional stress. *Cancer* **53**, 828-832.

Wellisch, D. K. and Yager, J. (1983) Is there a cancer-prone personality? *CA: Cancer J. Clin.* **33**, 145-153.

Wellisch, D. K., Jamison, K. R. and Pasnau, R. O. (1978) Psychosocial aspects of mastectomy II. The man's perspective. *Am. J. Psychiat.* **135**, 543-546.

Wenderlin, J. M. (1978) Women who have had mastectomy need increased social support: How do these women value mutual-support groups? In *Breast Cancer: Psychosocial Aspects of Early Detection and Treatment.* Brand, P. C. and van Keep, P. A., eds., pp. 9-14. University Park Press, Baltimore.

Wilson, J. F. (1981) Behavioral preparation for surgery: Benefit or harm? *J. Behav. Med.* **4**, 79-102.

Wirsching, M., Stierlin, H., Hoffman, F., Weber, G. and Wirsching, B. (1982) Psychological identification of breast cancer patients before biopsy. *J. Psychosom. Res.* **26**, 1-10.

Wirsching, M., Hoffman, F., Stierlin, H., Weber, G. and Wirsching, B. (1985) Prebioptic psychological characteristics of breast cancer patients. *Psychother. Psychosom.* **43**, 69-76.

Witkin, M. H. (1975) Sex therapy and mastectomy. *J. Sex Marital Ther.* **1**, 290-304.

Witkin, M. H. (1978) Psychosexual counselling of the mastectomy patient. *J. Sex Marital Ther.* **4**, 20–28.

Worden, J. W. (1983) Psychosocial screening of cancer patients. *J. Psychosoc. Onco.* **1**, 1–10.

Worden, J. W. and Weisman, A. D. (1980) Do cancer patients really want counselling? *Gen. Hosp. Psychiat.* **2**, 100–103.

Worden, J. W. and Weisman, A. D. (1984) Preventive psychosocial intervention with newly diagnosed cancer patients. *Gen. Hosp. Psychiat.* **6**, 243–249.

Youssef, F. A. (1984) Crisis intervention: A group-therapy approach for hospitalized breast cancer patients. *J. Adv. Nurs.* **9**, 307–313.

Zigmond, A. S. and Snaith, R. P. (1983) The Hospital Anxiety and Depression Scale. *Acta Psychiat. Scand.* **67**, 361–370.

Does Counselling by Nurses for Mastectomy Patients Work?

ROBERT CLACEY, CHRIS THOMAS and HENRY PEARSON

ABSTRACT

Twenty-five patients, who received counselling and education from a specially trained ward-based nurse, were compared with 25 mastectomy patients who received the educational elements alone. At 1 week after surgery the counselled patients were significantly less depressed on a variety of measures and had retained more educational information than the non-counselled patients. However, at 4 months there were no significant differences between the groups. Counselling for mastectomy patients is effective initially in relieving depression but there may be a need for continued counselling in order to maintain its effectiveness.

Myths and misconceptions about mastectomy and its effects are common, both within the public and amongst professionals. Renneker and Cutler in 1952 distinguished the psychological effects of having carcinoma of the breast from those of the mastectomy and concluded that it was the loss of the breast which engendered the primary emotional response. Some surgeons, however, have commented that the loss of the breast is a trivial event and psychological harm is a product of the investigation bias.

More scientific evidence of psychological disturbance after mastectomy has come from two sources – uncontrolled studies and controlled studies. The uncontrolled studies (Table 1) used such methods as postal questionnaires and advertisements in the media and this in part explains the wide variation in results, from 11% of mastectomy patients being psychologically disturbed in Lyons (1977) study to 83.5% in Torrie's (1970) study.

There have been two good controlled studies which provide more convincing evidence of the psychological ill-effects of mastectomy. Morris et al., (1977) conducted a 2 year follow-up study investigating 160 women under the age of 70 years presenting with a lump in the breast requiring biopsy. They obtained a group of 91 women with benign breast lumps and 69 women with breast carcinoma. The groups were not age-matched and the carcinoma group were on average 10 years older than the control group. A semi-structured interview was administered 1 day before biopsy and 3, 12 and 24 months later. The results showed that

159

TABLE 1. UNCONTROLLED STUDIES OF PSYCHOLOGICAL MORBIDY
FOLLOWING MASTECTOMY

		Psychological disturbance
Torrie	(1970)	83.5%
Roberts et al.	(1972)	50.0%
Winick and Robins	(1977)	13.0%
Lyons	(1977)	11.0%
Worden and Weisman	(1977)	20.0%
Jamieson et al.	(1978)	25.0%

25% of the mastectomy patients had failed to adjust at 2 years, they tended to be more depressed at each assessment on Hamilton rating scores and their sexual adjustment had deteriorated. The investigation questioned whether early intervention might reduce the psychological morbidity.

Maguire *et al.*, (1978) looked at psychiatric problems in the first year after mastectomy by comparing 75 women with carcinoma of the breast with 50 controls with benign breast disease. They administered a semi-structured interview pre-biopsy and at 4 and 12 months, to elicit depression, anxiety and sexual problems. The results showed that altogether 39% of the mastectomy patients had serious anxiety depression or sexual difficulties (compared with 12% of controls). In the mastectomy group eight women had sought help but only two thought that appropriate help had been given. Maguire concluded that "Inability to recognize and treat these emotional problems is a common and serious problem. Monitoring by specially trained nurses and social workers might help to identify them earlier and even reduce them." Given that psychological problems are a common complication of mastectomy what ways have been tried to help these patients? The following interventions have been suggested:

1. Multidisciplinary team support.
2. Post-mastectomy rehabilitation – multidisciplinary (Winnick and Robins, 1977).
3. Information services e.g. National Mastectomy Association (Bloom *et al.*, 1978).
4. Self-help groups e.g. those run by the Red Cross (Partridge and Thomas, 1985).
5. Ex-patient volunteer counsellors e.g. the Reach to Recovery programme in the U.S.A. (Martel, 1971).
6. Specially trained mastectomy nurse counsellors.

The effectiveness of any of these programmes is debatable. Only one properly controlled study has been undertaken. Maguire *et al.*, (1980) investigated the effectiveness of a special mastectomy nurse employed to see patients before surgery, 1 week after operation and then at home at least once and as often as needed thereafter. A trained interviewer assessed the psychiatric status shortly after surgery and at 3 months and 12-18 months. The results showed that altogether only 12% of counselled patients had appreciable anxiety or depression 12-18 months after mastectomy compared with 39% of non-counselled patients, this difference might not be due to nurse counselling but rather to the counsellor identifying and referring distressed women to a psychiatrist for treatment. With such limited evidence Morris' comment (1979) is still pertinent, "It is clear . . . that psychological morbidity from mastectomy exists, but its exact nature and amount, who suffers it, and whether it might be reduced are still only hinted at rather than convincingly demonstrated".

THE LEICESTER MASTECTOMY COUNSELLING SERVICE

Nurses on the surgical wards in Leicester felt that their mastectomy patients needed more psychological support and they discussed the option of employing a trained specialist nurse counsellor. The advantage of this would have been that one specialist with a lot of knowledge and experience would have been attached to the ward who could see mastectomy patients both before and after surgery, in the out-patients clinic, in hospital and afterwards at home. The disadvantages were that the specialist might not be considered to be fully part of the ward team, she might usurp the role of other nurses and that it would be an expensive option in a time of financial stringency.

The ward nurses in fact opted to allow three of their group to undergo training. They would then counsel mastectomy patients as part of their ordinary ward duties. The advantages were that these nurses would not be seen as outside specialists, that there would be a general improvement in counselling skills for the benefit of all patients, that the teaching of counselling skills to junior nurses on the ward would be improved and that no extra finances would be required. The major disadvantage of this choice was that the nurses could only see their patients whilst they were on the ward and they could not offer further help after discharge.

THE NURSE TRAINING PROGRAMME

The nurses chosen were one ward sister and two staff nurses and the following training programme was set up:

1. A lecture from a surgeon about surgical procedures and the provision of ample opportunity to ask questions about breast cancer and its treatment.
2. Two lectures from an oncologist-radiotherapist together with a

visit to the radiotherapy department and an opportunity to talk to radiotherapy nurses. They were also provided with photographs of the department and machines to show patients whilst in the ward so that they would have some awareness of what to expect during radiotherapy.

3. Meetings with surgical fitters from various prostheses firms to learn about fitting of temporary "comfy" prostheses as well as knowledge of the more permanent prostheses that would be available to the patients after discharge.

4. The nurses attended 10 seminars with a psychiatrist (CJT) and a social worker trained in counselling which covered such topics as goals of counselling, obtaining a contract, general listening skills, reactions to physical illness and talking through the reaction. The seminars involved a considerable amount of role-play. The nurses were also given guidance on how to recognize signs that might indicate serious psychiatric disturbance.

5. Once the nurses had started counselling mastectomy patients they received regular supervision of their counselling each week. The nurses counselled their patients in a room specially set aside for this purpose. It was furnished with comfortable chairs and a full length mirror to enable the counsellor to encourage the mastectomy patient to look at and touch her scar, and the appearance of a breast prosthesis once fitted. A full range of both temporary prostheses and permanent prostheses were kept in the counselling room so that they could be fitted by the same counselling nurse.

Counselling took place over the course of three interviews:—

First Interview (second or third day post-op)

The nurse facilitated discussion about how the woman felt about her operation, and the scar she had been left with. She was encouraged both to look at and touch the scar and to talk about her husband's attitude to it. The patient was shown (and again encouraged to touch) a temporary breast prosthesis which was then fitted. The nurse gently probed how much the patient knew about her diagnosis and would answer any question she was asked. It was suggested that the patient asks someone to bring in a well-fitting bra so that it could be tried on and discussed. If the bra fitted badly then it could be corrected prior to discharge.

On the 4th day post-op the nurse would give leaflets about local and national post-mastectomy services to the patient — one written by a woman who had a mastectomy.

Second Interview (fifth or sixth day post-op)

Talking again centred on how the woman was feeling, both physically and mentally. This led on to discussion about bone and liver scans, and the woman's knowledge about radiotherapy. Any fears the woman may have had about further treatment were aired. The nurse checked whether the woman had read the leaflets she had been given and whether they had found them to be helpful. Further discussion would take place about the diagnosis of breast cancer.

Third Interview (eighth or ninth day post-op)

The counselling nurse enquired about how the patient got on seeing the radiotherapist and ensured that she knew and understood all that he said. Plenty of opportunity was given for the patient to ventilate fears about radiotherapy. Going home was clearly an issue at this stage and ample time was available for the patient to discuss her feelings about discharge. The procedure for obtaining and fitting the permanent prosthesis was explained. Community services such as the National Mastectomy Association, a local shop selling special bras and clothes for mastectomy patients and the Red Cross medical aids service were introduced to the patient and explained. Finally the patient was advised what further avenues of help were available to her (e.g. G.P.) after discharge.

Each interview lasted approximately 45 min. and afterwards the nurse counsellor recorded accurately what had taken place during the interview with particular regard to the patient's emotional state. The counselling process is summarized in Table 2.

TABLE 2. FUNCTIONS OF LEICESTER WARD-BASED MASTECTOMY COUNSELLING SERVICE

1. Fitting of "comfy".
2. Discussion of prosthesis, bra and further treatment e.g. radiotherapy.
3. Information given re National Mastectomy Association
                Red Cross Self-Help Group
                Local shop for mastectomy products.
4. Ample time to discuss feelings re 1 to 3.
5. Supportive counselling (Rogerian style).

THE EFFECTIVENESS OF THE COUNSELLING SERVICE

When the nurse counselling service was in operation we were asked by the surgical team to assess its effectiveness. A simple pilot study was undertaken by asking the first 80 patients counselled by the nurses whether they were satisfied with the service they had been given. Seventy-five patients were satisfied and five dissatisfied. Of these five dissatisfied patients, three had profound psychiatric disturbance (two with a long-standing past psychiatric history) and needed referral to a psychiatrist, one was dissatisfied as her nurse counsellor became ill and she only received one counselling interview, and one patient was dissatisfied for reasons unknown.

The investigation proper was started in 1984. From Table 2 it can be seen that the service offered by the nurse counsellor to mastectomy patients in Leicester divides into two main components (1) an educational component (1-3) and (2) a counselling component (4-5). Following discussions with the surgical and nursing staff, it was felt to be unethical to withold information from mastectomy patients. We therefore aimed to assess the effectiveness of the ward-based nurse counselling service by comparing a group of women who received the educational component above (the non-counselled group) with a group who received both the educational and counselling elements of the service (the counselled group). The non-counselled patients were seen by the same nurses for about 20 min. They were instructed not to enter into discussion of feelings with these patients and to refer back any emotional questions to the surgical team.

All women referred to the counselling service with a mastectomy or sector mastectomy for carcinoma of the breast over a 6 month period were included in the study with the exception of cognitively impaired elderly women (three patients), and those unable to give consent (one patient). Alternative months in the study period were allocated to either counselling or non-counselling, and all patients admitted during that month were put in the appropriate group.

METHOD

The patients were assessed by a trained psychiatrist (RC) 1 week after surgery (where possible after the final counselling or non-counselling interview) and at home 4 months later. The initial post-operative semi-structured interview was used to obtain basic socio-demographic details, to assess the patient's knowledge of her illness and its treatment, her physical state and attitude to scar (using clearly defined operational criteria). The patient's knowledge of the post-mastectomy services and prostheses was noted in a similar way. The psychiatric status of the patient was assessed for anxiety and depression using a similar scale to that employed by Maguire et al., (1978) (i.e. 0, nil; 1, mild; 2, moderate; and 3, severe) at the time of interview and for each of the three preceding months to admission. The patient was asked to complete and return a Beck Depression Inventory (Beck et al., 1961), Spielberger's Anxiety Inventory (Spielberger et al., 1970), Crown Crisp Experiential Index (Crown and Crisp, 1979) and the General Health Questionnaire (Goldberg, 1979).

At the 4 month follow-up interview a further semi-structured interview took place. Further assessment was made of the patient's knowledge of illness, physical state and attitude to scar. As radiotherapy had been given, the patient's experience of this was noted, as was whether the patient had returned to work (if applicable) and the quality of the marital relationship and sexual adjustment (if relevant). They were asked about attendance at any post-mastectomy support services. Satisfaction with the "comfy" bra and permanent prosthesis was recorded. Psychiatric status for anxiety and depression at the time of interview and each of the months since discharge was assessed using the same scale as in the previous interview. The patients were given a Beck Depression Inventory, Spielberger State Anxiety inventory and General Health Questionnaire to return by post.

Twenty five counselled and 25 non-counselled patients completed the initial interview 1 week post-operatively. Of the counselled patients one refused the four month follow-up assessment and four others failed to return the postal questionnaires. Of the non-counselled patients three refused the four month follow-up assessment and three others failed to return the postal questionnaires. We were unable to detect any appreciable differences between those patients who completed all assessments and those who did not.

RESULTS

There were no significant differences between the counselled and non-counselled groups with regard to age, marital status, past psychiatric history, time between the woman discovering her breast lump and presentation to G.P., and whether the woman had a sector or a full mastectomy.

From Table 3 it can be seen that on the basis of the psychiatric state scales the counselled patients are significantly less depressed than the non-counselled patients ($P < 0.01$). However, there was a trend for the non-counselled patients to have been more depressed in the 3 months prior to surgery, raising the question of whether the results are biased in favour of the counselled group.

There was no difference between the two groups in terms of anxiety either at interview or in the 3 months prior to surgery. The questionnaire results 1 week after surgery supported these findings (Table 4). The counselled group were significantly less depressed on the mean Beck

TABLE 3. DEPRESSION AND ANXIETY ONE WEEK AFTER SURGERY — BY PSYCHIATRIC STATE SCALES

	C (n = 25)	NC (n = 25)	
Mod–Severe Depression in 3 month pre-op period	5	10	
Mod–Severe Depression on interview	0	7	$P < 0.01$
Mod–Severe Anxiety in 3 month pre-op period	11	10	
Mod–Severe Anxiety on interview	4	5	

TABLE 4. QUESTIONNAIRE RESULTS ONE WEEK AFTER SURGERY

	C (n = 25)	NC (n = 25)	
Beck Depression Inventory score (mean)	3.8	8.8	$P < 0.01$
Beck "cases" (score 14 +)	0	6	$P < 0.03$
Crown–Crisp Index – depression scale	3.5	5.3	$P < 0.05$
Spielberger–State Anxiety score (mean)	33.6	37.8	
General Health Questionnaire score (mean)	4.2	6.5	

TABLE 5. MODERATE—GOOD KNOWLEDGE OF TREATMENT AND POST-MASTECTOMY SERVICE ONE WEEK AFTER SURGERY

	C (n = 25)	NC (n = 25)	
Radiotherapy	9	1	$P < 0.01$
Temporary prosthesis	16	8	$P < 0.05$
Red Cross Service	9	4	
National Mastectomy Association	8	2	
Local Mastectomy shop	7	4	
Permanent prosthesis	17	11	

TABLE 6. DEPRESSION AND ANXIETY 4 MONTHS AFTER SURGERY — BY PSYCHIATRIC STATE SCALES AND QUESTIONNAIRES

	C	NC
Mod–Severe depression at interview	11	13
Mod–Severe anxiety at interview	8	10
Beck score (mean)	5.6	8.8
GHQ score (mean)	4.5	6.84
Spielberger-State score (mean)	32.4	38.3

score ($P < 0.01$) and in terms of number of Beck "cases" ($P < 0.03$) using a cut-off score of 14, which Beck recommends to indicate caseness, and the depression scale of the Crown–Crisp Experiential Index ($P < 0.05$). There was also a non-significant trend for the non-counselled group to score higher on the Spielberger-State Anxiety score and the General Health Questionnaire. On all scores the counselled patients had better knowledge of treatment and post-mastectomy support services than non-counselled patients, 1 week after surgery (Table 5) although, only Radiotherapy and Temporary Prosthesis were statistically significant. The counselled group had significantly better knowledge of radiotherapy and the temporary prosthesis and tended to have better knowledge of the Red Cross self-help service, a local mastectomy shop and the permanent prosthesis. In addition to this the counselled group had significantly better acceptance of their scar with only five of the 25 counselled patients being judged to have difficulty accepting the scar compared with 14 of the 25 non-counselled patients ($P = <0.02$). Table 6 indicates various scores for anxiety and depression 4 months after surgery. There were no significant differences between 24 counselled patients and 22 non-counselled patients in depression or anxiety as assessed at the interview.

CONCLUSIONS
There were a number of shortcomings with this study:
1. Relatively small sample size.
2. The use (for ethical reasons) of a control group who received part (the educational component) of the nurse counselling service rather than an ideal control group who received none of the service. The counselling nurses may have inadvertently been drawn into certain counsellor functions or given the factual information in different ways to each group.
3. The time differences between the control group interviews (about 20 min each session) and the counselling interviews (about 45 min each session). Were the differences between the groups a result of a non-specific factor of spending more time with the counselling nurse rather than a specific effect of the counselling itself?
4. The trend for the non-counselled group to have been more depressed in the 3 months prior to surgery raises the question of bias in favour of the counselled group. However, this assessment of depressed mood was made retrospectively and may have been exaggerated by the current depressed mood in the non-counselled group.
5. The absence of any pre-operative assessment.

Despite these shortcomings we were encouraged that our findings support to an extent Maguire et al's, study (1980). Counselling results in a mastectomy patient having a better attitude towards her scar, better knowledge of her temporary prosthesis, and, initially, a lower level of depression. The improvement in depression was not maintained at 4 months. Counselling appears to have no impact on anxiety, either initially or at 4 months. The benefits of counselling are largely lost at 4 months. One disadvantage of a ward-based nurse-counselling service is that the counsellor is unable to follow-up the patient after discharge. Perhaps if they were able to offer this follow-up the benefits of counselling would be maintained.

REFERENCES

Beck, A. T., Ward, C. H., Mendelson, M., Mock, J. and Erbaugh, J. (1961) An inventory for measuring depression. *Arch. Gen. Psychiat.* **4**, 561–571.
Bloom, J. R., Ross, R. D. and Burnell, G. M. (1978) The effect of social support on patient adjustment following breast surgery. *Patient Counsel. Health Educ.* **1**, 50–59.
Crown, S. and Crisp, A. H. (1979) *Manual of the Crown–Crisp Index.* Hodder & Stoughton, London.
Goldberg, D. P. (1979) *Manual of the General Health Questionnaire.* NFER-Nelson Windsor.
Jamison, K. R., Wellisch, D. K. and Pasnau, R. O. (1978) Psychosocial aspects of mastectomy: I. The woman's perspective. *Am. J. Psychiat.* **135** (4), 432–436.

Lyons, J. S. (1977) Breast Cancer Management Early and Late. Stoll, B. A., ed., Heinemann Medical, London.

Maguire, G. P., Lee, E. G., Bevington, D. J., Kuchemann, C., Crabtree, R. J. and Cornell, C. E. (1978) Psychiatric problems in the first year after mastectomy. Br. Med. J. 1, 963–965.

Maguire, G. P., Tait, M., Brooke, M., Thomas, C. J. and Sellwood, R. (1980) Effect of counselling of the psychiatric morbidity associated with mastectomy. Br. Med. J. 281, 1454–1456.

Martel, W. M. (1971) The American Cancer Societies programme for the rehabilitation of a breast cancer patient. Cancer 28, 1676–1678.

Morris, T., Greer, H. S. and White, P. (1977) Psychological and social adjustment to mastectomy: a 2-year follow up study. Cancer 40, 2381–2387.

Morris, T. (1979) Psychological adjustment to mastectomy. Cancer Treat. Rev. 6, 41–46.

Partridge, S. and Thomas, C. J. (1985) Mastectomy Self-Help Group. Effects of attendance on psychosocial outcome after surgery, in press.

Renneker, R. and Cutler, M. (1952) Psychosocial problems of adjustment to cancer of the breast. J. Am. Medi. Assoc. 148, 833–839.

Roberts, M. M., Furnival, S. G. and Forrest, A. P. M. (1972) The morbidity of mastectomy. Br. J. Surg. 59, 301–302.

Spielberger, C. D., Gorsuch, R. L. and Lushene, R. E. (1970) Manual for the State-trait Anxiety Inventory. Consulting Psychologists Press, Palo Alto, California.

Torrie, A. (1970) Like a bird with broken wings. Wld Med. April 7, 36–47.

Winnick, L. and Robins, G. F. (1977) Physical and psychologic readjustment after mastectomy. Cancer 39, 478–486.

Worden, J. W. and Weisman, A. D. (1977) The fallacy in post-mastectomy depression. Am. J. Med. Sci. 273 (2), 169–175.

Psychotherapeutic Interventions for Cancer Patients Treated with Chemotherapy

ABSTRACT

Chemotherapy is a complex type of cancer treatment which produces a wide range of side effects. Certain side effects, such as anticipatory nausea and vomiting can be treated successfully with psychotherapy. Also, for some patients, chemotherapy is so intolerable that they do not complete it. However, the responsibility for discontinuation may evoke psychological morbidity, so that psychotherapy is indicated. Two case reports are described to illustrate the use of psychotherapy with these types of problem.

Until recently, psychotherapy was exclusively for distressed people who were unable to deal with their problems, but a new awareness of the extent of psychological morbidity in cancer patients has led to the use of psychotherapy for those whose life has been changed by cancer. The survival rate of cancer patients has now increased significantly (Cullen, 1981; DeVita, 1982) and psychotherapy should be given high priority as a form of treatment for patients who are unable to cope with the consequences of this disease.

Because psychotherapeutic oncology is a relatively new area and few systematic data are available, clinical case reports and clinical research should be performed and published to promote the development of psychotherapeutic oncology on a larger scale. Therefore, two case reports are presented with patients of different ages and with different problems related to cancer treatment, which illustrate different psychotherapeutic interventions and processes.

CASE 1: SIDE EFFECTS OF CHEMOTHERAPY

Chemotherapy treatments affect the quality of life of patients severely. Such treatments may last from 1 to 2 years and produce a wide range of side effects, the most disturbing and frequently encountered being nausea and vomiting (Sallin and Cronin, 1982; Nerenz et al., 1982), which usually occurs *after* administration of the drug. The stress is characterized mainly by feelings of helplessness, personal failure,

169

despair and (latent) anger (Cohn, 1982; Brinkley, 1983). However, it is less widely known that nausea and vomiting can also occur *before* the administration of such drugs (Redd and Andrykowski, 1982; Morrow and Morrell, 1982) and that these anticipatory effects increase in frequency and severity with increasing duration of the treatment (Cotanch, 1983).

Research has shown that anticipatory nausea and vomiting (AN/V) occur mildly in 25-45% of patients (Redd, 1984) and severely in 10 to 15% (Altmeier *et al.*, 1982) and a number of authors have explained this in terms of acquired or conditioned responses. Repeated association of chemotherapy with the unwanted reactions can lead to triggering of the response by formerly neutral situations, such as catching sight of the hospital or smelling the cytostatic agents. It has also been assumed that patients who are susceptible to AN/V have an inhibitive coping style.

The results of psychotherapeutic treatment for nausea and vomiting following chemotherapy have not been encouraging (Catanch, 1983; Lyles *et al.* 1982), but more success has been reported for this form of treatment with respect to nausea and vomiting preceding chemotherapy (Redd and Andrykowski, 1982; Morrow and Morrell, 1982).

The first patient was a 57-year old, robust, pleasant woman with two grown-up children. Her husband had retired from a responsible position. She underwent amputation of the right breast for carcinoma, a pneumectomy for lung metastasis, and chemotherapy (CMF) was indicated by a chest radiograph suggesting tumour tissue behind the heart. After four courses of CMF the patient developed symptoms of AN/V which increased in intensity and duration. After the fifth course she was referred by her oncologist for psychotherapy (Bos-Branolte and Cleton, 1985).

Treatment

For obvious reasons, the psychotherapy was performed at the therapist's home rather than in the hospital. During the first few sessions the problems were analysed to distinguish between treatment related and non-treatment related aspects, in other words, anxiety on the one hand and inhibitive coping style and lack of coping skills on the other. At the same time, a start was made with the treatment plan which consisted of: progressive muscle relaxation (PMR), systematic desensitization (SD), guided imagery, modelling or learning-by-imitation method, and psychodynamic methods.

The following example will serve to illustrate this approach to deeper-lying conflicts. During the patient's frequent fits of crying, the therapist confronted her with questions about feelings she might be avoiding by crying. This makes it possible to "disclose" feelings and thus release a pathway for direct expression. During the fourth and last session at home, the patient expressed long suppressed feelings of anger, indignation, disappointment and grief. Resentment against her husband to whom she always gave in, against her daughter who had criticized her for going to talk with "someone else", against her elderly mother who was critical of her because she vomited, against her family doctor who wanted to prescribe Valium, against her friends who visited her in the hospital when she had a broken leg but almost none of whom came when her breast was amputated, and against her family, who maintained the classically unhelpful projection that it is better for her not to talk. And lastly, resentment against herself for accepting all this and not standing up for herself.

Just as she reached the door, the patient confessed that during chemotherapy treatments she became incontinent and had to be thickly diapered. She was deeply ashamed of this and had never told anyone about it before.

I mention this range of accusations and complaints to illustrate another point as well: That cancer is always a social problem too.

After four sessions of 45 min each at home, one session was held in the Department of Clinical Oncology to complete psychotherapeutic treatment.

Psychotherapeutic treatment of AN/V in this patient was extremely effective. The treatment consisted of four sessions in the therapist's home followed by one session at the Department of Medical Oncology. The first four sessions were partially successful: she was able to keep the nausea and vomiting under control from the day before the chemotherapy through the seeing and entering of the hospital. The second part of the psychotherapy — before and during the administration of the chemotherapy — had complete and persistent results. The symptoms were completely under control during all of the subsequent courses, which meant that the patient was free of nausea and vomiting both prior to, and during, each of the last four courses. Moreover, the patient was in complete remission.

Detailed retrospective analysis of the circumstances which gave rise to the vomiting during chemotherapy showed that, at least for this patient, classical conditioning is an oversimplified explanation of AN/V, since this symptomatic behaviour is also triggered by increasing anxiety for, and lack of coping skills, in the stress situation itself. Furthermore, it became clear that, from the clinical point of view, AN/V has two components, one occurring well in advance of the medical treatment (from 1 day before to just before it is started) and the other *during* the medical treatment, including the period of waiting.

CASE 2: COMPLIANCE WITH CHEMOTHERAPY

Compliance with drug treatment is a problem in many branches of medicine but is not widely recognized as such in clinical oncology (Redd *et al;* 1982). A review of the National Surgical Adjuvant Breast Project Study performed in the U.S.A. showed that about 30% of the patients failed to complete 2 years of treatment (Morrow and Morrell, 1982). However, discontinuation of treatment may result in feelings of guilt, anxiety, uncertainty and isolation and even in suicidal attempt as will be illustrated in the second case report of a gynaecologic cancer patient.

The patient was 25 years old when ovarian carcinoma, 'stage 1C, was diagnosed. She underwent radical bilateral adnexa extirpation and abdominal uterus extirpation, which made her infertile and menopausal. After surgery, chemotherapy was indicated. However, during the first of the six prescribed courses of chemotherapy, the patient discontinued the treatment.

The consequences were rather dramatic. She developed claustrophobia and relational and sexual problems. This resulted in physical deterioration, because she was blamed for being the cause of her cancer. After a suicidal attempt she needed professional help and was referred for psychotherapy.

Treatment

The treatment plan consisted of: progressive muscle relaxation (PMR), guided imagery, psychodynamic therapy, partner relation therapy, and sex therapy.

In the psychotherapeutic sessions, a great deal of time was spent on the question of why she had discontinued chemotherapy; her motives were rather vague and it appeared to be a heavy responsibility. It was not until after several sessions that she became aware of her need for control and her inability to accept or ask for medical support, perhaps partly because she was a nurse.

After she left the hospital, she did not leave her home for months because of hair loss. Her friends saw her as rational and strong, but remembering this period she said: "I didn't want to be different, but they did not see beyond the surface". In fact, she felt deserted. Moreover, she had never been sick before and it made her feel ashamed and she also felt it as unfair. Gradually, she obtained more insight into her own behaviour.

The relationship with her partner had deteriorated too. On the one hand, she thought she no longer had anything to offer him, since she was infertile and menopausal now, but on the other hand she blamed him for their not having tried to have children some years earlier. She deplored the loss of her smooth belly and was disgusted by the big scar and the pendulous skin around it. Relation therapy and sex therapy were both started. Her partner, who felt exhausted too, learned to communicate about his problems and to negotiate about his needs. For both of them, the infertility gave rise to serious emotional problems. After coping with cancer, coping with infertility had to be worked through. The constant discussion of *in vitro* fertilization in the mass media stimulated them to fantasize about it, which was a severe obstacle to coping with it. Finally, they decided to wait for another year and to cope with their old problems instead of creating new ones.

The sessions took place over a period of 1 year, in the beginning once a week, later twice a month. During psychotherapy, the patient gradually learned to improve her coping skills and after several sessions together with her partner, the partner relationship and the sexual relationship improved considerably. Finally, she decided to resume her medical treatment and was found to be free of cancer.

At follow-up sessions 6 and 12 months after the end of the psychotherapy, the positive gains from psychotherapy were stabilized and extended. It can therefore be concluded that, in this case, psychotherapy resulted in compliance with medical treatment and improved the quality of life for both the patient and his partner.

In both cases described psychotherapy distinctly improved the coping skills of oncology patients. These patients seem to learn more quickly and selectively than general (non-cancer) clients and are more eager to improve the quality of their life.

REFERENCES

Altmeier, E. M., Ross, W. E. and Moor, K. (1982) A pilot investigation of the psychologic functioning of patients with anticipatory vomiting. *Cancer* **49**, 201-204.
Bos, G. (1983) Effects of gynaecological cancer on the quality of life of young women. In Proceedings of the 5th EORTC Study Group on Quality of Life October 6-8, 1983, Leiden, The Netherlands.
Bos-Branolte, G. and Cleton, F. J. (1985) Psychotherapie ter behandeling van bijwerkingen van chemotherapie. *Med. Contact* **40**, 1493-1495.
Brinkley, D. (1983) Emotional distress during cancer chemotherapy. *Br. Med. J.* **286**, 663-664.
Cohn, K. H. (1982) Chemotherapy from an insider's perspective. *Lancet* **i**, 1006-1009.
Cotanch, P. (1983) Relaxation training for control of nausea and vomiting in patients receiving chemotherapy. *Cancer Nurs.* **6**, 277-283.
Cullen, J. W. (1981) Research issues in psychosocial and behavioral aspects of cancer. *Proc. Am. Cancer Soc.* 157-164.
DeVita, V. T. Jr. (1982) Statement to the 13th International Cancer Congress, Sept. 1982, Seattle, U.S.A.
Lyles, J. M., Burish, T. G., Krozely, M. G. and Oldham, R. K. (1982) Efficacy of relaxation training and guided imagery in reducing the adversiveness of cancer chemotherapy. *J. consul. Clin. Psychol.* **50**, 509-524.
Moher, D., Arthur, A. Z. and Pater, J. L. (1984) Anticipatory nausea and/or vomiting. *Cancer Treat. Rev.* **11**, 257-264.
Morrow, G. R. and Morrell, C. (1982) Behavioral treatment for the anticipatory nausea and vomiting induced by cancer chemotherapy. *New Eng. J. Med.* **307**, 1476-1480.
Nerenz, D. R., Leventhal, H. and Love, R. R. (1982). Factors contributing to emotional distress during cancer chemotherapy. *Cancer* **50**, 1020-1027.
Redd, W. H. (1984) Behavioral interventions for control of treatment of side effects . In *Current Concepts of Psycho-Oncology* pp. 53-54, Memorial Sloan Ketting Centre, New York.

174 *Gerjanne Bos*

Redd, W. H. and Andrykowski, M. A. (1982) Behavioral intervention in cancer treatment: Controlling aversion reactions to chemotherapy. *J. Consult. Clin. Psychol.* **50**, 1018-1029.

Redd, W. H., Rosenberger, P. H. and Hendler, C. S. (1982) Controlling chemotherapy side effects. *Am. J. Clin. Hypnosis* **25**, 161-172.

Sallan, S. E. and Cronin, C. M. (1982) Nausea and Vomiting. In *Cancer Principles and Practice of Oncology.* DeVita, V. T., Hellman, S., Rosenberg, S. A.. eds., 1704-1707. J. B. Lippincott, Philadelphia/Toronto.

Schain, W. S. (1981) Role of the sex therapist in the care of the cancer patients. In J. M. Vaeth *et al.*, eds. *Pharmaceutical Aspects of Cancer Care. Front. Radiat. Ther. Oncol.* **15**, 168.

Is Cancer Nursing Stressful or Satisfying?

SUSIE WILKINSON

ABSTRACT

The paper focuses on a recent study of stressors and satisfiers in cancer nursing. Eighty-eight nurses working in two cancer hospitals completed self administered questionnaires, and tape-recorded interviews were also carried out with ten randomly selected nurses.

Results are discussed in terms of the most satisfying and stressful experiences encountered by the nurses, to whom the nurses felt they could turn for support, whether the support offered was perceived as adequate and the areas of work where nurses felt inadequately prepared to carry out their role.

It has been well established that nursing is a profession with high levels of stress (Vachon, 1978; Chiriboga et al., 1983; Hodgkinson, 1984). Clearly, over the last decade, stress in nursing has captured the attention of researchers from a variety of disciplines. Most studies have focused on intensive care units (Koumans, 1965; Hay and Oken, 1972; Huckabay & Jagla, 1979; Claus and Bailey, 1980) but in recent years studies in America have focused their attention on the causes of stress among nurses working with cancer patients.

The results of these studies have been strikingly different in terms of both whether cancer nursing is inherently stressful, and also the primary stressors experienced by nurses, which have included the long and protracted and unpleasant treatments patients receive (Kane, 1984), the severing of a lengthy relationship by the death of a patient causing the nurse a real sense of loss (Vachon, 1978), the role conflicts between doctors and nurses (Oberst, 1980; Lederberg, 1982), the mutilating surgery patients were subjected to (Lederberg, 1982), the work overload (Doovan, 1981), the lack of psychological support from peers and the presence of a bureaucratic organizational structure with the hospital (Yasko, 1983).

Apart from one study (Murgatroyd and Hitch, 1984), only anecdotal accounts as to the causes of stress were identified in the U.K. literature. Furthermore, there appeared to be a paucity in both the American and British literature on the sources of satisfaction in cancer nursing.

It seemed pertinent to try to identify the sources of stress and satisfaction among British nurses working with cancer patients. As cancer is the second largest cause of death in Britain (OPCS, 1982) most nurses throughout their careers will be responsible for the care of cancer patients. It is well recognized that the effects of stress on an individual reduces their level of work performance, causes ill health and dissatisfaction and results in higher absenteeism and turnover of staff, situations clearly to be avoided in the present cutbacks occurring in our National Health Service. On the other hand individuals who feel satisfied with their work are likely to feel more contented, do a better job and be less likely to leave (Baron and Byrne, 1981).

The Aims of the Study were to identify:

1. The most satisfying and stressful situations experienced by nurses working with cancer patients in two cancer hospitals.
2. The similarities and differences in both satisfying and stressful situations between nurses in each hospital.
3. To whom nurses relate their satisfying and stressful situations.
4. To whom within the hospital the nurse felt she could turn for support.
5. Whether the nurses perceive the support offered to be adequate.
6. Any area of work where the nurses did not feel they had been sufficiently prepared to carry out their role.

METHOD

The data were collected by administration of a self-report questionnaire containing closed and open questions and incorporating the critical incident technique (Flanagan, 1954). Critical incidents are specific events described by individuals as having significant meaning to them. Tape recorded interviews were undertaken with 10 randomly selected nurses. Answers to the closed questions were coded ready for computation. Answers to the open-ended questions were categorized using content analysis. The tape recorded interviews were rated, categorized, transcribed and re-rated.

The Sample

The sample consisted of 88 registered and enrolled nurses working in two specialist cancer hospitals (one in the north and one in the south of England) who had at least 4 months experience as a permanent member of staff working on any ward or department except the children's wards or theatres.

The two groups of nurses were equally matched in terms of positions held (Figure 1).

RESULTS

Using the χ^2 Test at 0.05 significance level, it was found that there were significant differences between the nurses from Hospitals A and B.

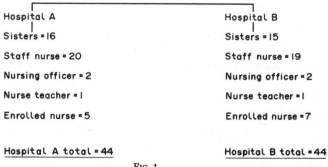

Sample
N = 88

Hospital A
Sisters = 16
Staff nurse = 20
Nursing officer = 2
Nurse teacher = 1
Enrolled nurse = 5

Hospital A total = 44

Hospital B
Sisters = 15
Staff nurse = 19
Nursing officer = 2
Nurse teacher = 1
Enrolled nurse = 7

Hospital B total = 44

FIG. 1.

TABLE 1. RELIABILITY STUDY FOR
CATEGORIZATION OF SATISFYING AND
STRESSFUL INCIDENTS

Satisfying incidents	Agreement
Rates 1 vs Rater 2	0.8835
Rater 1 vs Rater 3	0.8835
Rater 2 vs Rater 3	1.000
Stressful incidents	
Rater 1 vs Rater 2	1.000
Rater 1 vs Rater 3	0.9471
Rater 2 vs Rater 3	0.9471

Firstly, nurses from Hospital B had been qualified longer than nurses from Hospital A — $P < 0.05$. Secondly more nurses were married at Hospital A than at Hospital B but were slightly younger —$P < 0.07$, not quite reaching the level of statistical significance. Thirdly, significantly more nurses (42), had undertaken the ENB course in oncology nursing at Hospital B compared to nurses (11) from Hospital A, $P < 0.0001$.

A reliability study was carried out between three raters and Cohen's Kappa coefficients indicated that levels of agreement reached were satisfactory (Table 1).

Sources of Stress

Seventeen categories of stress emerged from the data (Table 2). From these 17 categories, those relating to similar areas of stress were combined to form five main categories and these were:
   (i)   conflicts with health care workers;
   (ii) communication difficulties with patients and relatives;

TABLE 2. STRESSFUL INCIDENTS FOR NURSES

Sub Category	Frequency of Incidents	% of Incidents
Nurse/Doctor conflicts	28	17.0
Inability to communicate effectively with patient	16	9.5
Threatening to self-comfort/safety (psychological)	14	8.3
Difficulties with communicating and supporting relatives regarding treatments/bereavements	13	7.8
Inability to give adequate care due to staff shortage/lack of time	13	7.8
Death of young patients or of similar age to nurse	11	6.5
Not carrying out nursing care to the required standard due to own mistakes/judgements	9	5.3
Unexpected sudden death of patient	9	5.3
Conflicts with paramedics/ancillary staff	7	4.2
Watching patients' conditions deteriorate	7	4.2
Stress resulting from policies implemented by nursing administration	7	4.2
Being unable to carry out terminal care of patients through to the end	7	4.2
Nursing patients with uncontrolled pain	6	3.5
Being assessed (exams, interviews, appraisals)	6	3.5
Lack of support and guidance from members of the nursing staff	6	3.5
Nurse felt she had insufficient knowledge to deal with situation	47	2.3
Personal conflicts with own ward staff	5	2.9
Total number of incidents	168	100

(iii)   deterioration and death of patients;

(iv)   poor care;

(v)   personal stresses.

1. *Conflicts with health care workers.* Although nurses recorded conflicts involving nursing colleagues, paramedic and ancillary staff, in this category overall "Conflicts with doctors", was the major source of stress in this study, as illustrated by the following example.

"When a young patient died following chemotherapy, who in my opinion should not have had treatment as he was dying anyway, I could not see or agree with the medical staff's rationale for treating him and nor could his wife and I have to pick up the pieces after he died, which was not easy. I felt bad in that I couldn't explain to the patient's wife why the doctor did it."

Twenty two out of the 28 nurse/doctor conflicts recorded were related to the doctors' prescription of chemotherapy or analgesia, which in the nurses' views were often prescribed inappropriately. Nurses' views and opinions regarding patients' treatments were rarely sought in this study, even though they were responsible for nursing the patients 24 hours a day. The data from the 10 nurses interviewed revealed some ambivalence in their relationships with doctors. Six nurses maintained their relationships were good and supportive whereas four nurses expressed severe dissatisfaction in their relationships with doctors. These four were all staff nurses and made the following kind of comment: "They're not approachable, only interested in the sisters, not staff nurses, they treat us like children."

This raised the question of whether it was only the staff nurses who had recalled stressful incidents in the nurse/doctor category? This was not confirmed, as only 10 out of the 28 incidents were recalled by staff nurses. This suggests that all grades of nursing staff can experience such conflicts.

2. *Communication difficulties with patients and relatives.* Seventeen percent of the stressful incidents recalled were in this category and were related to nurses indicating that they did not know how to handle questions which patients and relatives had posed. Not only did nurses find communicating with patients and relatives stressful but 65% of nurses described patients, relatives and colleagues as the most difficult areas of their work. When asked about areas of their work where they felt they needed further training, 51% of nurses wrote communication/ counselling skills. This was of particular interest, as 60% of the nurses in the study had completed the ENB course in oncology nursing which includes communication skills in the curriculum.

3. *Deterioration and death of patients.* The largest difference between the nurses in the two hospitals occurred in this category (Hospital A 28 incidents, Hospital B 11 incidents). This was important as few nurses at Hospital A had completed the ENB course in oncology nursing which covers care of the dying patient. This seems to suggest that extra education in this area may help nurses come to terms with nursing dying patients whereas inadequate preparation could be an exacerbator of stress.

The evidence indicated that death alone was not a source of stress, the stress arose when it was an unexpected death, a young death, or a patient of the same age as the nurse. This supports Glaser and Strauss's (1964) finding that nurses are particularly moved when the patient's death is a grave "social loss". When the nurses were stopped from completing this area of care because patients were transferred to other hospitals, hospices or their homes to die, the nurses were stressed. This may have been because they felt guilty or cheated about not being able to carry out care to the end.

4. *Poor care.* All the incidents in this category were related to the nurses inability to give the patients the nursing care they believed to be appropriate. In the main this was due to shortages of staff which resulted in a lowering of standards and risk taking (when nurses were expected to deal with situations with insufficient knowledge). There were no differences between the nurses from each hospital in the recall of incidents in this category.

TABLE 3. SATISFYING INCIDENTS FOR NURSES

Sub Category	Frequency of Incidents	% of Incidents
Carrying out and seeing positive results from nursing procedures (physical)	23	13.4
Giving support to patients through interaction with them	21	12.2
Nursing dying patients and supporting their grieving relatives	18	10.5
Receiving visits from ex-patients or hearing from them (showing improvement)	14	8.1
Receiving positive remarks from fellow members of the health care team	11	6.5
Being accepted for/appointed to nursing post of choice	11	6.5
Seeing a patient discharged home	11	6.5
Organizing something different/special for patients	10	5.9
Helping patients through a course of chemotherapy	10	5.9
Personal growth/development, courses/learning	9	5.2
Being thanked by relatives/patients	9	5.2
Being in charge of a ward when everything runs smoothly	8	4.7
Feeling needed	7	4.1
Nursing patients when they are no longer in pain	5	2.9
Hearing of or being with patients when they are told they are disease free	4	2.4
Total number of incidents	171	100

5. *Personal stresses.* The sub-categories making up this category were related to the nurses being assessed, examined or feeling threatened by those around them.

Sources of Satisfaction

Fifteen sub-categories emerged from the data (Table 3) and those relating to similar areas of satisfaction were combined to form three main categories:
(i)   caring for patients;
(ii) receiving positive reinforcements; and
(iii) personal developments.
1. *Caring for patients.* This was shown to be the major satisfier in this study, supporting the findings of Hockey (1976). This result was not unexpected considering all the nurses involved in the study had completed their general training and had opted to remain in a profession whose particular function was to care for people.

The most important sub-category was carrying out and seeing positive results from nursing procedures.

The second sub-category, "giving support to patients through interaction with them", illustrated that nurses who felt able to talk to patients openly gained a lot of satisfaction from such interactions.
2. *Receiving positive reinforcement.* Obtaining explicit positive reinforcement by receiving thanks or visits from patients and fellow

health care workers and by witnessing patients' improvements and discharges, was the second main category of incidents recalled by the Registered nurses whereas for the Enrolled nurses this main category of incidents provided the *most* important source of satisfaction.

One reason for the slight inconsistency with the Registered nurses may be due to the more vulnerable position of Enrolled nurses, in that they are considered second level nurses and feelings of recognition may be more important to enhance their satisfaction, particularly at this present time when their future is under threat. But overall, this result is a forceful reminder of how important it is to be able to say thank you or offer words of praise or encouragement to all grades of staff. Something many of us find so hard to do but something that obviously can have an effect on how contented a nurse can feel with her job.

3. *Personal development.* The incidents in this category were mainly related to gaining promotion, attending conferences and further education, which demonstrates how vital opportunities for post basic education may be in sustaining satisfaction in nursing.

Overall only three nurses were unable to recall the two satisfying incidents asked for, which suggests that most nurses in this study were quite satisfied with their jobs.

Support for nurses

The nurses were asked if they felt supported by their nurse managers. Sixty-three (72%) believed they were. Even accepting that questionnaires can produce answers which the respondents believe the investigator will want to hear (Hockey, 1976), this seems to be convincing evidence that nurses in this study felt supported. The nurses were also asked about the levels of support they received. Fifty-four percent felt the level of support being offered was satisfactory, 46% felt they would like more support than was currently being given and no-one indicated that they wanted less support. There was considerable agreement between the nurses from both hospitals over support.

Overall job satisfaction

On Hockey's (1976) assumption that individuals who feel satisfied with their job would choose the same job again if given the chance, the nurses were asked if they would choose to nurse cancer patients again. Ninety-five percent of nurses stated they would choose the same job again. Even allowing for the idea that people tend to give favourable answers when asked how they liked their job, (Blauner, 1960, Goldthorpe *et al.*, 1970) this response is convincing evidence that nurses in this study were experiencing a high degree of job satisfaction.

DISCUSSION

The evidence from this study suggests that poor communication between the nurses and doctors is a possible cause of the conflicts experienced. The nurses appeared to feel dominated by the doctors. As situations which are externally controlled are often perceived as highly stressful (Lefcourt, 1974) the domination itself could be considered the source of stress. It is suggested that nurses may need to improve their communication skills if they are to avoid further conflicts. The nurse/doctor relationship certainly needs nurturing as there is a growing body of evidence which demonstrates that good relationships and communications can have a positive effect on patient care and patient outcome. (Knaus et al., 1986).

Poor communication skills also caused stress for nurses while caring for patients. Maybe some nurses do enjoy talking to patients and their relatives, but from the stresses recorded and the requests for further help in this area, it has to be concluded that the nurses did not feel very competent at handling the awkward questions or situations they encountered.

The stress reported could be due to the nurses knowingly distancing themselves from patients (Maguire, 1985). Such behaviour can prevent patients from talking about their problems and the nurses may have felt stressed by their guilt at being unable to help patients. Further research is indicated in order to clarify this suggestion. However, there is evidence from this study to indicate that the present ENB course in oncology nursing may not be adequately preparing nurses in this area.

Despite the stresses involved, a very large proportion of the nurses in the study were obviously able to cope with the stresses as most had worked with cancer patients for an average of 4½ years whereas one study found that nurses rarely stayed in oncology nursing for longer than 3 years, because of the high levels of burn-out experienced in the speciality (Stewart et al., 1982).

The interviews conducted with 10 of the nurses proved valuable in revealing several factors that could have been responsible for the high levels of job satisfaction the nurses enjoyed.

Firstly, the hospital atmosphere/environment. The nurses consistently referred to the *different* ward and hospital atmospheres and claimed it was less stressful and much more satisfying to nurse cancer patients in their present environment than in general hospital wards.

A formal, regimented environment, where more emphasis is placed on "getting through the work" (Clarke, 1978), where patients are nursed in closed-awareness contexts (Glaser and Strauss, 1966) and where staff relationships are hierarchical, increases the amount of stress experienced by nurses caring for cancer patients.

Secondly, the nurses indicated that if they had a satisfying personal relationship and a good social life, they felt more able to cope with the stresses of the job, and were less likely to take their work worries home with them. This supports Prophit's (1981) observation that good personal relationships prevent nurses from becoming over-committed, a characteristic that has been described as rendering a nurse more vulnerable to burn-out.

The majority of nurses said they had not experienced signs of burn-out, while working in their present positions, enough to warrant them having any time off or feel as if they did not want to come to work, although two nurses reported having felt like that during their general training. Sleep disturbances, periods of anxiety and crying lasting longer than 2 days were reported by only one nurse who admitted nursing cancer patients had caused her such distress she had just handed in her resignation.

Thirdly, the high levels of job satisfaction could have arisen because those who chose to nurse cancer patients may have already established, in their general training, whether or not they could cope with the specific difficulties the work entails.

Overall, it was concluded that although the results of the study cannot be generalized because of the small sample, there was substantial evidence to suggest that nurses working in these two specialized hospitals did not find nursing cancer patients inherently stressful. This is contrary to the findings of several American studies (Kane, 1984; Yasko, 1983; Lederberg, 1982) but the results do indicate that caring for cancer patients in general hospital wards may be problematic and is an area worthy of further investigation.

REFERENCES

Baron, R. and Byrne, D. (1981) *Social Psychology: Understanding Human Interaction*, 3rd ed. Allyn & Bacon, Boston.
Blauner, R. (1960) Work satisfaction and industrial trends in modern society. In Galenson, W. and Lipset, S. M., eds., *Labour and Unionism*. John Wiley, New York.
Chiriboga, D., Jenkins, C. Bailey, J. (1983) Stress and coping among hospice nurses: test of an analytic model. *Nurs. Res.* 32(5), 294–299.
Clarke, M. (1978) Getting through the work. In Dingwall, R. and McIntosh, J., Ed., *Readings in Sociology*. Livingstone, Edinburgh.
Claus, K. E., Bailey, J. T. (Eds) (1980) *Living with Stress and Promoting Well-being*. C. V. Mosby Co., St. Louis.
Donovan, M. I. (1981) Stress at work: cancer nurses report. *Oncol. Nurs. Forum* 8(2), 22–25.
Flanagan, J. C. (1954) The critical incident technique. *Psychol. Bull.* 51, 327–358.
Glaser, B. and Strauss, A. (1964) The social loss of dying patients. *Am. J. Nurs.* 64(6), 119–121.
Glaser, B. and Strauss, A. (1966) *Awareness of Dying. A Sociological Study of Attitudes Towards the Patient Dying in Hospital*. Weidenfeld & Nicolson, London.
Goldthorpe, J. H., Lockwood, D., Beckhofer, F. and Platt J. (1970) *The Affluent Worker: Industrial Attitudes and Behaviour*. Cambridge University Press, Cambridge.
Hay, D. and Oken, D. (1972) The psychological stresses of intensive care unit nursing. *Psychosom. Med.* 34, 109–118.

Hockey, L. (1976) *Women in Nursing*. Hodder & Stoughton, London.

Hodgkinson, P. (1984) Nursing stress. *Nurs. Times*, **Oct 10**, 33-36.

Huckabay, L. M. D. and Jagla, B. (1979) Nurses' stress factors in the intensive care unit. *J. Nurs. Admi.* **9**(2), 21-26.

Kane, N. E. (1984) How to make cancer nursing more bearable. *Reg. Nurs.* **47**, 45-47.

Knaus, W. A., Draper, E., Wagner, D. and Zimmerman, J. (1986) An evaluation of outcomes from intensive care in major medical centres *Ann. Intern. Med.* **104**, 410-418.

Koumans, A. H. R. (1965) Psychiatric consultations in an intensive care unit. *J. Am. Med. Assoc.* **194**, 163.

Lederberg, M. (1982) Support groups/stress in oncology. Proceedings of a symposium at Memorial-Sloan Kettering Cancer Centre. *Curr. Concepts Psychosoc. Oncol.* 89-91.

Lefcourt, H. (1974) Locus of control and acceptance of one's reinforcement experience. *Colloquia* 204.

Maguire, P. (1985) Barriers to psychological care of the dying. *Br. Med. J.* **291**, 1711-1713.

Murgatroyd, J. and Hitch, P. (1984). Professional problems investigated. *Nurs. Mirror*, **159**(4), 36-37.

Oberst, M. T. (1980) Research highlights: a study in cancer control. *Cancer Nurs.* **3**(5), 384.

Office of Population Censuses and Surveys (1982) *Cancer statistics*. HMSO, London.

Prophit, P. (1981) Burnout. The cost of involvement of being human in the helping professions. *Research a Base for the Future*. 403-406. University of Edinburgh Nursing Studies, Edinburgh.

Stewart, B., Meyerowitz, B., Jackson, L. Yarkin, K. and Harvey, J. (1982) Psychological stress associated with out-patient oncology nursing. *Cancer Nurs.* 383.

Vachon, M. L. (1978) Motivation and stress experienced by staff working with the terminally ill. *Death Educa.* **2**, 113-122.

Yasko, J. M. (1983) A survey of oncology clinical nursing specialists. *Onco. Nurs. Forum*, **10**, 25-30.

E.   Terminal Illness

Quality of Death from Lung Cancer: Patients' Reports and Relatives' Retrospective Opinions

S. AHMEDZAI, A. MORTON, J. T. REID and R. D. STEVENSON

ABSTRACT

The relatives of 40 patients who died of lung cancer were interviewed by a research nurse and social worker, who had previously assessed the "quality of life" from the time of diagnosis to death in the same patients. Relatives were asked about the patients' symptoms, mood state, awareness of disease and problems met in the last month of life. Their opinions revealed important differences from the patients' own reports. The commonest terminal problems recalled were "pain", "loss of independence" and "weakness". Fifty seven per cent of the patients died in hospital: of these, 20% had been unwilling to be admitted there for terminal care.

Studies of the quality of life in cancer patients tend to focus on the early stages of disease, when active oncological treatments are applied, in order to evaluate the toxicity of therapy as well as the relief of symptoms (Selby, 1985). It is equally important to examine the terminal stages of cancer in these patients, not least because many current treatment protocols have been shown to leave long term physical and emotional side-effects (Aisner and Wierwek, 1982; McArdle et al., 1981). Knowledge of the specific problems encountered by patients and relatives during terminal disease would also be invaluable in planning appropriate health care supportive services (Cartwright, 1983).

There is natural reluctance to subject terminally-ill patients to exhaustive questionnaires or interviews, particularly if they are not familiar with the research team and methods of study. An alternative source of information on the problems of terminal illness has therefore been the relatives' retrospective opinions, sought many months after bereavement (Cartwright et al., 1973). Applied uncritically, this method may give incomplete or misleading information about the experiences during life. We wished to examine the validity of the retrospective approach, by comparing the bereaved relatives' opinions with the patients' own reports before death.

METHOD

We have conducted (Ahmedzai et al., 1984) a cohort study of lung cancer patients from the time of diagnosis to death, in which monthly interviews and questionnaires applied by a research nurse and social worker recorded the symptoms, mood and awareness of disease, as well as other variables of "quality of life". The same research assistants contacted by letter, and arranged to interview the nearest relative (or close friend) of the patients after death. Selection of patients and relatives was strictly sequential; only if it was known that a patient had not had close contact with another person during the last months of life was he excluded from study. Forty-one relatives were approached and one declined to participate. The time elapsed since death was <6 months for 7% of cases, 6–12 months for 53%, 12–18 months for 33% and 18–24 months for the remaining 7%. All interviews were conducted in the relatives' homes, and lasted from 1 to 3 hours.

At the interview, relatives were asked to report on the patients' illness, by answering identically worded questions on symptoms and mood selected from the patients' questionnaires. Mood was assessed by means of the Leeds General Scales for Anxiety and Depression (Snaith et al., 1976). They were also asked about the patients' insight into their diagnosis and prognosis. Finally, the relatives were asked to comment on the problems affecting the patients during the last month of life, especially relating to hospital admission. Because the "retrospective" questionnaires were completed by the research assistants, there were very few items omitted or unevaluable. Previous testing had shown good correlation between the two assistants' scoring for such questions.

RESULTS

Symptoms in last month of life

Four of the commonest symptoms reported by the lung cancer patients were "dyspnoea", "anorexia", "pain" and "constipation". Table 1 shows a comparison of the mean scores for each of these symptoms, between the patients' own ratings and their relatives' retrospective opinions. All of the symptoms were rated slightly higher by the relatives than by the patients. The correlation (Spearman's r) of scores between the groups was below the level of significance for all but "dyspnoea". The reason for this lack of correlation being observed in spite of not too dissimilar mean scores, is the lack of agreement of individual pairs of scores from the two sources, leading to a wide scatter of scores as demonstrated in the example of "pain".

Mood in last month of life

In Table 2 the mean scores for five of the items from the Leeds Anxiety and Depression General Scales, obtained from patients and relatives are compared. One item, "Frightened/panic" yielded the same mean score in

TABLE 1. SYMPTOMS IN LAST MONTH OF LIFE: CORRELATIONS BETWEEN PATIENTS' OWN AND RELATIVES
RETROSPECTIVE REPORTS

| | Mean Score (0 = best/3 = worst) | | r | P |
	Patients	Relatives		
Dyspnoea	1.4	1.8	0.56	<0.01
Appetite	1.8	1.9	0.26	NS
Pain	1.9	2.0	0.24	NS
Constipation	1.4	2.0	0.24	NS

TABLE 2. MOOD IN LAST MONTH OF LIFE: CORRELATIONS BETWEEN PATIENTS' OWN AND RELATIVES
RETROSPECTIVE REPORTS

| | Mean Score (0 = best/3 = worst) | | r | P |
	Patients	Relatives		
Miserable/sad	2.0	1.5	0.36	NS
Life not worth living	1.2	0.6	0.32	NS
Early wakening	1.9	1.5	0.22	NS
Irritable	2.0	1.6	0.25	NS
Frightened/panic	0.9	0.9	0.22	NS

both groups. For the other four items, namely "Miserable/sad", "Life is not worth living", "Early wakening", and "Irritable", the relatives consistently scored lower than the patients. There was no significant correlation observed for any of these items once again because of the individual pairs of relative and patient often giving widely different scores.

Insight into disease

In Table 3 the relatives' and patients' own reports on awareness of disease (Diagnosis and Prognosis) are compared. Regarding the grades of insight into "Diagnosis" shown, the term "Full insight" is used to indicate that the patient explicitly stated that he knew he had lung cancer; "Partial insight" means that he showed by his words or actions that he was incompletely aware, e.g. he suspected but had not been told; "Wrong" indicates that he believed that he was suffering from another disease, e.g. pneumonia. The relatives' ratings suggest that they believed more patients had fuller insight into the diagnosis of lung cancer than the patients themselves indicated, or wished to indicate to the research staff during their last month of life. The difference in grades of awareness was not significant when analysed by χ^2 test.

With regard to awareness of "Prognosis", the term "Terminal" here indicates that the patient believed that he would certainly die as a result of his disease; "Very serious" means that he felt his life was likely to be at risk; "Serious" that he thought death was a possibility but unlikely; "Not serious" that he fully expected a complete recovery, or no risk to his life.

TABLE 3. AWARENESS OF DISEASE IN LAST MONTH OF LIFE: COMPARISON OF PATIENTS' OWN AND RELATIVES' RETROSPECTIVE REPORTS.

	% Patients	% Relatives	χ^2
Insight into diagnosis —			
Full insight	40	89	
Partial insight	50	11	4.0
Wrong	0	0	(NS)
Don't know	10	0	
Insight into prognosis —			
Terminal	55	82	
Very serious	18	9	
Serious	18	0	2.9
Not serious	0	9	(NS)
Don't know	9	0	

The results show that, as with insight into "Diagnosis", relatives tended to report more frequently an awareness of imminent death, than the patients had personally conveyed. Once again the differences were not statistically significant.

Problems encountered in terminal illness

The commonest problems in the month before death, according to the relatives were: "Pain" (47.5%); "Loss of independence" (37.5%); "Weakness" (30%); "Anorexia" (27.5%); "Anxiety", "Breathlessness" and "Constipation" (each 12.5%). Thirty three per cent of patients had three symptoms or problems in the month before death, 19% had four symptoms and 6% had five symptoms.

Death occurred at home for 35%, in hospital for 57.5%, in a hospice for 5% and on holiday for one patient. Admission to hospital had occurred at least 2 weeks prior to death in 16%, between 1–2 weeks in 12%, less than 1 week in 52% and less than 24 hours in 20%. The relatives recalled that 20% of patients had been "very keen" on hospital admission, 20% "agreeable", 20% "equivocal", 16% "reluctant" and one patient had been admitted against his expressed wishes. The relatives themselves had been left with "positive" feelings about hospital admission in 76% of cases, and "negative" feelings in 20% (one relative was equivocal). The reasons precipitating admission were: "Weakness" (64%), "Pain" (52%), "Confusion" (28%), "Mood disorder", "Respiratory" and "Gastrointestinal" symptoms (each 16%).

DISCUSSION

It was only possible to conduct this study because we had previously carried out a prospective evaluation of quality of life in patients with lung cancer. This gave us the material with which to compare the retrospective opinions of bereaved relatives and close friends. The additional fact that the research workers were well known to the subjects probably increased the numerical yield of data, although it is acknowledged that some bias could also have possibly arisen from this acquaintance.

The discrepancies between the patients' and relatives' scores on symptom and mood items from the questionnaire are interesting. It is not clear why the relatives consistently scored symptoms higher, and mood items lower than the patients had done. It would be premature to conclude from these limited data that any major systematic bias must exist in the recall or perception of relatives, although it is quite likely that with the passage of time, their memories do become distorted. The results indicate that it would be fruitful to conduct a larger study to examine the sources and extent of such bias, and to assess whether it is influenced by the severity of the patients' illness, or the relatives' own coping abilities.

The differences observed between the relatives' opinions and the patients' own reports of their awareness of disease, although not statistically significant in this sample, suggest the need for caution in adopting without reservation, retrospective data on this important subject. It is extremely difficult to obtain reliable information from patients about their insight into disease processes and prognosis, and even more so to attempt categorization of their comments and non-verbal responses (Hinton, 1980). It is probable that in their last weeks of life, the patients under study may have considerably understated (i.e. "denied") their disease, or the research workers may have underestimated their subjects' statements. Alternatively, it may have been difficult for the relatives to dissociate their own level of knowledge from their memories of the patients' awareness. Once again, we consider it important to repeat this aspect of the study in a larger group, and to examine how the communication within couples during life, and even the length of time since death, may influence subsequent recall of awareness.

The brief data presented here on the relatives' views of the problems in the last month of life carry potentially important implications for the provision of health care to terminal cancer patients and their families. It is noteworthy that "loss of independence" and "weakness" followed "pain" as the commonest problems experienced, and the "weakness" even preceded "pain" as the commonest reason for hospital admission. The finding that only 40% of patients had been actively willing to go into hospital for terminal care, and 20% had been admitted unwillingly underline the need for increasing the scope and number of community-oriented terminal care systems, such as the specialist nursing services and home-based symptom control teams.

In conclusion, this small study has revealed the necessity to look critically at the use of data gathered retrospectively from relatives, on the terminal stages of cancer. Larger studies are required to confirm the findings and to evaluate further the problems of dying from other forms of cancer. Such research may also produce new insights into bereavement reactions. It would be useful, we believe, if research into "quality of life" which is being actively pursued in cancer clinical trials were extended into the "quality of death", with an emphasis on psychosocial as well as physical problems.

ACKNOWLEDGEMENTS

This research was supported by a grant from the Chest, Heart and Stroke Association (Scotland).

REFERENCES

Ahmedzai, S., Reid, J. T., Morton, A. and Stevenson, R. D. (1984) Effects of chemotherapy on quality of life in patients with lung cancer. (Abs.). *Thorax* **39**, 719.

Aisner, J. and Wiernek, P. H. (1982) Complications of treatment and of improved survival in patients with small cell carcinoma of the lung, 1, 381–398. In Greco, *et al.*, eds. *Small Cell Lung Cancer.* Grune & Stratton, New York.

Cartwright, A. (1983) *Health Surveys in Practice and in Potential.* King's Fund, London.

Cartwright, A., Hockey, L. and Sanderson J. L. (1973) *Life Before Death.* Routledge & Kegan Paul, London.

Hinton J. (1980) Whom do dying patients tell? *Br. Med. J.* **281**, 1328–1330.

McArdle C. S. (1981) The social, emotional and financial implications of adjuvant chemotherapy in breast cancer. *Br. J. Surg.* **68**, 261.

Selby, P. (1985). Measurement of the quality of life after cancer treatment. *Br. J. Hosp. Med.* **33**, 266–271.

Snaith, R. P., Bridge, G. W. and Hamilton, M. (1976) The Leeds Scales for the self-assessment of anxiety and depression. *Br. J. Psychiat.* **128**, 156–165.

Depression Among Cancer Patients Admitted for Hospice Care

JENNIFER HUGHES AND DEBORAH LEE

ABSTRACT

The prevalence of depressive symptoms among patients with advanced cancer, admitted to a hospice, was assessed with the Hospital Anxiety and Depression Scale. Of a total of 50 patients, 13 (26%) had severe depression and 6 (12%) of the 50 were receiving antidepressant treatment. Associations between depression and various organic and psychological factors are discussed.

Patients with advanced cancer may be depressed for a number of reasons:
1. Reactive to the illness:
   (a) distressing physical symptoms;
   (b) unwanted effects of anticancer treatments;
   (c) knowledge of impending death.
2. Due to organic brain syndrome:
   (a) cerebral metastases;
   (b) metabolic abnormalities e.g. hypercalcaemia, hepatic failure;
   (c) drug effects.
3. Coincidental, e.g. other recent adverse life events or social difficulties, past history of recurrent depression.

Previous work (Plumb and Holland, 1977; Bukberg et al., 1984; Derogatis et al., 1983) shows that approximately a quarter of patients in hospital with advanced cancer of various types have definite clinical depression: if borderline cases are included the proportion is roughly half. There are a limited number of systematic studies on the topic, and we suggest there are three main reasons which make investigation difficult:
1. There is an overlap between "pathological" depressions which merit treatment, and appropriate "depressive reactions" which some consider an inevitable, even desirable, stage in the process of adjusting to fatal illness.
2. There is an overlap between the somatic symptoms of depressive illness and the symptoms of advanced cancer, making diagnosis difficult. Both conditions frequently cause anorexia, weight loss, constipation, loss of energy, insomnia, pain and general malaise.

193

3. Many professionals are diffident about raising emotionally charged issues with patients who have incurable cancer. They fear questioning will be perceived as an intrusion, or that it will precipitate an outpouring of distress for which there is no remedy. For patients who are very weak or in pain, any interview which is done for research purposes rather than because it has direct relevance to individual clinical care may seem difficult to justify.

Despite these problems it seems important to examine our knowledge about mood disorder in such patients. Severe depression in those dying of cancer is not the norm, and it may be possible to prevent or treat the condition in the minority who are vulnerable.

The present study was done in Countess Mountbatten House, our local continuing care unit for cancer patients. Patients come from three health districts; Southampton, Portsmouth and Winchester. Only about 60% of admissions to the unit end in the patient's death, the other 40% end in discharge home after satisfactory relief of pain, vomiting, or other specific symptoms which necessitated admission. Besides the inpatients, the unit has a caseload of outpatients receiving domiciliary care. We realize that these inpatients form a small, selected sample of the total population of those with advanced cancer in the area concerned, so our findings cannot be generalized to those at home or in other hospitals.

METHOD

All patients admitted to the unit during a 3-month period were considered for the study, but of 87 consecutive admissions there were 36 who were already moribund and could not take part. Only one refused. Fifty patients (16 men, 34 women) were interviewed. Their ages ranged from 36 to 85 with a mean of 63. A variety of primary tumour sites was involved. Our interviews lasted on average 30–40 min., (which still proved too long for some patients to finish), and covered the following topics:

(a)   sociodemographic details;
(b)   pain;
(c)   mood;
(d)   past psychatric history;
(e)   religion;
(f)   satisfaction with information given about illness;
(g)   worst part of illness;
(h)   greatest comfort during illness; and
(i)   other major life events during year.

Three rating scales were used:
  (i)   Hospital Anxiety and Depression (HAD) scale (Zigmond & Snaith,

1983): a selfrating instrument which consists of psychological, rather than somatic, symptoms of mood disorder.
(ii) Minimental state: a simple test of cognitive function (Folstein *et al.*, 1975).
(iii) Karnofsky scale: a 10-point scale to measure the amount of activity the patient can manage (Karnofsky, 1968).

RESULTS

In relation to mood, about a quarter of patients said they felt very depressed indeed, most of the time, half said they sometimes got depressed, and the remaining quarter said they were not depressed at all. The depressed patients all considered their physical illness was the main reason for their depression, even if they reported other stresses such as a recent bereavement.

On the HAD depression subscale, 13 patients scored as definitely depressed, six as borderline and 31 as not depressed. Although we were not able to validate this scale against a full psychiatric interview, the scores appeared to correspond quite well with clinical state. A few patients who did appear depressed at interview obtained low scores, whereas one item on the scale — "I feel as if I am slowed down" — extracted a false positive response from several patients whose weakness and retardation appeared physical rather than mental.

Six of the whole group were taking tricyclic antidepressants on admission. They included three severely depressed patients.

The search for correlates of depressed mood was unrewarding in that none of the factors we examined proved to have a statistically significant association with it. Some of the trends which emerged were rather surprising, though with a sample of only 50 patients, such trends might be due to chance. For example: depression was more often found in the men than the women; it was less common in younger patients; it was less common in patients with a past psychiatric history: it was less common in patients with known cerebral metastases; it was more common in those who were living with relatives, presumably because those who lived alone or in institutions had nobody close to worry about; it was less common in those who had been widowed or divorced, presumably for the same reason; and it was not associated with nearness to death. Other trends were in the expected direction, for example depression was more common in patients who were in pain, who had cognitive impairment, who were physically dependent, who lacked a strong religious belief, and who were not well-informed about their illness.

We looked at these last two factors in a little more detail. For religion, 18 patients had a strong faith, 14 said they did believe but this was not of great importance to them, and 16 were atheist or agnostic. Thirteen patients said their religious belief had become stronger since they had been ill, and two had changed from Church of England to a different faith (Roman Catholicism and Spiritualism respectively). Only two said their faith was weaker. Though the religious patients did derive comfort from their faith, a substantial number were nevertheless depressed.

Patients' knowledge of their illness was not simple to classify. We did not ask direct questions about "cancer" and a number of patients obviously wanted to avoid discussing the topic. The well informed patients were less likely to be depressed than the rest.

Those who were sufficiently robust to complete the interview were asked to name the worst aspect of the illness, and also what had been their greatest comfort. By far the most frequent worst aspect was the forced inactivity, and the most frequent comfort was the support of family and friends.

In conclusion, this study suggests that between a quarter and a third of cancer patients, admitted to a continuing care unit, are clinically depressed and that many depressed patients have not been given a trial of antidepressants before admission, either because their depression was not recognized, or because it was assumed to be untreatable.

As a closing comment, nearly all patients seemed pleased to take part in the study and found the questions acceptable and the medical student interviewer (DL), despite some initial trepidation, found carrying out this work a rewarding experience which was of clear value in her medical training.

REFERENCES

Bukberg, J., Penman, D. and Holland, J. C. (1984) Depression in hospitalised cancer patients. *Psychosom. Med.* **46**, 199–212

Derogatis, L. R., Morrow, G. R., Fetting, J., Penman, D., Piasetsky, S., Schmale, A. M., Henrichs, M. and Carnicke, C. L. M. (1983) The prevalence of psychatric disorders among cancer patients. *J. Am. Med. Assoc.* **249**, 751–757.

Folstein, M. F., Folstein, S. E. and McHugh, P. R. (1975) Mini-mental state. *J. Psychiat. Res.* **12**, 189–198.

Karnofsky, D. A. (1968) Clinical evaluation of anticancer drugs. In Golden, A. ed., *Cancer Chemotherapy.* Japanese Cancer Association, Tokyo.

Plumb, M. M., and Holland, J. (1977) Comparative studies of psychological function in patients with advanced cancer — I. Self reported depressive symptoms. *Psychosom. Med.* **39**, 264–276.

Zigmond, A. S. and Snaith, R. P. (1983) The hospital anxiety and depression scale. *Acta Psychiat. Scand.* **67**, 361–370.

Stress in Home-Care and Hospital Support Nurses for the Terminally Ill

JACKIE YARDLEY and BARRY LUNT

ABSTRACT

Working with the dying has been shown to be stressful to nurses in a wide range of specialities. Hospice nurses may be vulnerable to burn-out because of their constant exposure to death.

We studied 37 English home care and hospital support teams for the terminally ill. One hundred and six nurses and their managers were asked about sources of stress. Relationships with professional colleagues were cited by 55% of nurses and demands on time by 32%. Fifty-four per cent mentioned some aspect of patient or family care, but no one aspect was cited by over 20%. Death and bereavement were mentioned by only 29%, for 14% this was in relation to young people. Sources of stress were related to the age of the service, and the nurses' age and qualification in terminal care, but not to their community experience, terminal care experience, or whether they felt they had enough support.

These findings indicate that professional relationships are seen as stressful by more nurses than are the issues of death and dying.

Index

options discussion 123
and quality of life 65, 66
uncertainty 123
Career, view of cancer patients 26
Cervical cancer, attitudes 127
Cervical smear test, impact of
    abnormal 127, 128
Chemotherapy
  adjuvant
    assessments 102, 103
    impact after mastectomy 101-11
    regime 102
    survival rates 101
    trial design 102
  adverse effects 105, 107, 108, 122
  duration 169
  compliance study 171, 172
  conditioned reflex symptoms 105, 107
  depressive effects 104-6, 108
  emotional distress 109
  patients' opinions 107
  psychological morbidity 97, 121
  psychotherapy 169-73
Children and psychological morbidity 98
Circulatory system, mortality after
    widow(er)hood 36
  interval 38, 39
CMP (cyclophosphamide, methotrexate
    and 5-fluorouracil)
  emotional distress 108, 109
  psychological cost 109
Colposcopy 127
Communication
  hospital 81
  nurse: doctor 178, 179, 182
  uses 77, 78
Complementarity principle 84
Compliance, chemotherapy 171, 172
Conditioned reflex symptoms 105, 107
Coping
  bone marrow transplantation 6-10
  children 13, 14
  emotion-focused 18
  and hospitalization 17, 18
  leukaemia 13-20
  motor disturbances 16, 17
  psychotherapy 173
  quality of life 67
  school, post-treatment 18, 19
  style, manuals 140
Coping strategies 19
  adolescents 13
  assessment 58
  life-events and cancer 57
Courtauld Emotional Control Scale 141,
    142
  breast cancer 141, 142, 148
Crown-Crisp Index, mastectomy

counselling 166

Danish Cancer Registry 54
Delay, presenting breast lumps 72, 73
Denial, cancer 46, 47
Depression
  cancer patient in hospice 193-6
    drug use 195
  cancer progression 57, 58
  causes 193
  chemotherapy 104-6, 108
  informed patients 196
  investigation problems 193
  post-mastectomy 121, 122, 146-8, 165
    counselling 166
    treatment 104-6
  pre-mastectomy 141, 142, 165
  rating scales 194, 195
  treatment discussion 123, 124
Diagnosis
  delay and stress 122, 123
  discussion over 153
  lessening impact 124, 125
  pejorative 152
  psychological consequences 119-26
  psychological morbidity 93, 94
  uncertainty 123

Effort after meaning phenomenon 55

Family, stress buffer 18, 19
Fight, cancer 46, 47
Frontal lobe defect 15

General Health Questionnaire
  mastectomy 102
    counselling 166
    post-, treatments 105, 106
Genetic disorders 7
Global evaluation of life 63
Graft-vs-host disease 4

Hair loss 98, 108
Helplessness/hopelessness in cancer 46,
    47
  altering 48
  sex 49
Home care, stress 197
Homeostatic controls and cancer 57
Home tutors, cancer treatment 25, 26
Homogamy 34
  and mortality of spouse 38
Hopelessness
  measurement 49
  and outcome 49
Hospice care
  cancer patient depression 193-6
  patient features 194, 195